Working to overcome the global impact of neglected tropical diseases

First WHO report on neglected tropical diseases

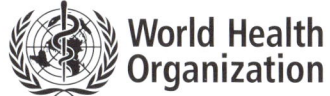

WHO Library Cataloguing-in-Publication Data

First WHO report on neglected tropical diseases: working to overcome the global impact of neglected tropical diseases.

    1 Tropical medicine - trends. 2 Endemic diseases. 3 Poverty areas. 4. Parasitic diseases. 5 Developing countries. 6. Annual reports. I. World Health Organization

ISBN 978 92 4 1564090   (NLM Classification: WC 680)

Working to overcome the global impact of neglected tropical diseases was produced under the overall direction and supervision of Dr Lorenzo Savioli (Director, WHO Department of Control of Neglected Tropical Diseases) and Dr Denis Daumerie (Programme Manager, WHO Department of Control of Neglected Tropical Diseases), with contributions from staff serving in the department.

Regional directors and members of their staff provided support and advice.

Valuable inputs in the form of contributions, peer reviews and suggestions were received by members of the Strategic and Technical Advisory Group for Neglected Tropical Diseases.

The report was edited by Professor David W.T. Crompton, assisted by Mrs Patricia Peters.

© World Health Organization 2010

All rights reserved. Publications of the World Health Organization can be obtained from WHO Press, World Health Organization, 20 Avenue Appia, 1211 Geneva 27, Switzerland (tel.: +41 22 791 3264; fax: +41 22 791 4857; e-mail: bookorders@who.int). Requests for permission to reproduce or translate WHO publications – whether for sale or for noncommercial distribution – should be addressed to WHO Press, at the above address (fax: +41 22 791 4806; e-mail: permissions@who.int).

The designations employed and the presentation of the material in this publication do not imply the expression of any opinion whatsoever on the part of the World Health Organization concerning the legal status of any country, territory, city or area or of its authorities, or concerning the delimitation of its frontiers or boundaries. Dotted lines on maps represent approximate border lines for which there may not yet be full agreement.

The mention of specific companies or of certain manufacturers' products does not imply that they are endorsed or recommended by the World Health Organization in preference to others of a similar nature that are not mentioned. Errors and omissions excepted, the names of proprietary products are distinguished by initial capital letters.

All reasonable precautions have been taken by the World Health Organization to verify the information contained in this publication. However, the published material is being distributed without warranty of any kind, either expressed or implied. The responsibility for the interpretation and use of the material lies with the reader. In no event shall the World Health Organization be liable for damages arising from its use.

Design, layout and figures: Denis Meissner, Claudia Corazzola, Christophe Grangier, WHO/GRA.
Unless otherwise stated, all maps and photographs were produced by WHO.

Printed in France
WHO/HTM/NTD/2010.1

Contents

Foreword by the Director-General   iii

Executive summary   vii

PART 1

1. **Neglected tropical diseases: a paradigm shift**   1
   - 1.1 Common features of neglected tropical diseases   2
   - 1.2 New strategic approaches   2
   - 1.3 Refocusing   3
   - 1.4 Lessons learnt   4

2. **Sixty years of growing concern**   7
   - 2.1 World Health Assembly resolutions   8
   - 2.2 Landmarks in prevention and control   8
   - 2.3 Strategic and Technical Advisory Group for Neglected Tropical Diseases   10

3. **Human and economic burden**   13
   - 3.1 Epidemiological burden   13
   - 3.2 Economic burden   15
     - 3.2.1 Economic impact   15
     - 3.2.2 Costs of interventions   17

4. **Ways forward**   21
   - 4.1 Approaches to overcoming neglected tropical diseases   21
     - 4.1.1 Preventive chemotherapy   22
     - 4.1.2 Intensified case-management   25
     - 4.1.3 Vector control   26
     - 4.1.4 Safe water, sanitation and hygiene   28
     - 4.1.5 Veterinary public health: zoonotic aspects of neglected tropical diseases   28
   - 4.2 Current policies and strategies   29
     - 4.2.1 The *Global plan to combat neglected tropical diseases 2008–2015*   31
     - 4.2.2 Neglected tropical diseases and the Millennium Development Goals   32
     - 4.2.3 Neglected tropical diseases and health-system strengthening   34

PART 2

5. Neglected tropical diseases in the world today — 39
- 5.1 Dengue — 41
- 5.2 Rabies — 47
- 5.3 Trachoma — 55
- 5.4 Buruli ulcer (*Mycobacterium ulcerans* infection) — 59
- 5.5 Endemic treponematoses — 64
- 5.6 Leprosy (Hansen disease) — 69
- 5.7 Chagas disease (American trypanosomiasis) — 75
- 5.8 Human African trypanosomiasis (sleeping sickness) — 82
- 5.9 Leishmaniasis — 91
- 5.10 Cysticercosis — 97
- 5.11 Dracunculiasis (guinea-worm disease) — 103
- 5.12 Echinococcosis — 107
- 5.13 Foodborne trematode infections — 113
- 5.14 Lymphatic filariasis — 117
- 5.15 Onchocerciasis (river blindness) — 123
- 5.16 Schistosomiasis (bilharziasis) — 129
- 5.17 Soil-transmitted helminthiases — 135

6. Global and regional plans for prevention and control — 143
- 6.1 Health targets — 143
- 6.2 Regional plans — 146

7. Conclusions — 147
- Overcoming neglected tropical diseases: 7 gains, 7 challenges — 149

Annexes — 153
1. Resolutions of the World Health Assembly on neglected tropical diseases — 155
2. Official list of indicators for monitoring progress on the Millennium Development Goals — 159
3. Summary of metadata — 163
4. Methods used to prepare maps and charts — 169

Available in electronic format
WHO's global and regional plans for prevention and control
- African Region
- Region of the Americas
- Eastern Mediterranean Region
- South-East Asia Region
- Western Pacific Region

Foreword
by the Director-General of the World Health Organization

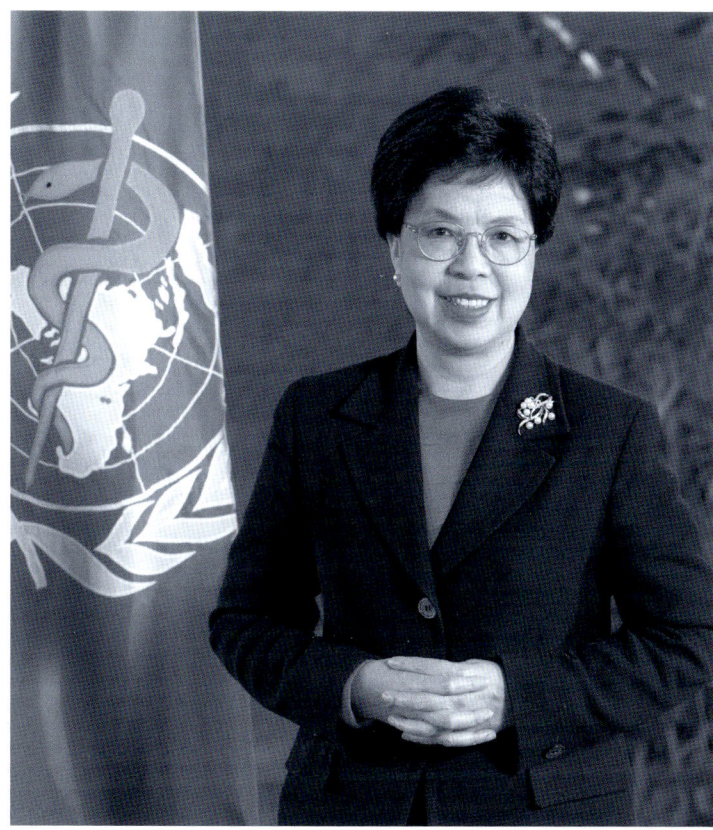

Tackling neglected tropical diseases: a pro-poor strategy on a grand scale

Though medically diverse, neglected tropical diseases form a group because all are strongly associated with poverty, all flourish in impoverished environments and all thrive best in tropical areas, where they tend to co-exist. Most are ancient diseases that have plagued humanity for centuries.

Once widely prevalent, many of these diseases gradually disappeared from large parts of the world as societies developed and living conditions and hygiene improved. Today, though neglected tropical diseases impair the lives of an estimated 1 billion people, they are largely hidden, concentrated in remote rural areas or urban slums and shantytowns. They are also largely silent, as the people affected or at risk have little political voice.

Neglected tropical diseases have traditionally ranked low on national and international health agendas. They cause massive but hidden and silent suffering, and frequently kill, but not in numbers comparable to the deaths caused by HIV/AIDS, tuberculosis or malaria. Tied as they are to impoverished tropical settings, they do not spread to distant countries and only rarely affect travellers as, for example, during outbreaks of dengue. Because they are a threat only in impoverished settings they have low visibility in the rest of the world. Though greatly feared in affected populations, they are little known and poorly understood elsewhere. While the scale of the need for prevention and treatment is huge, the poverty of those affected limits their access to interventions and the services needed to deliver them. Diseases linked to poverty likewise offer little incentive to industry to invest in developing new or better products for a market that cannot pay.

Today, neglected tropical diseases have their breeding grounds in the places left furthest behind by socioeconomic progress, where substandard housing, lack of access to safe water and sanitation, filthy environments, and abundant insects and other vectors contribute to efficient transmission of infection. Close companions of poverty, these diseases also anchor large populations in poverty. Onchocerciasis and trachoma cause blindness. Leprosy and lymphatic filariasis deform in ways that hinder economic productivity and cancel out chances for a normal social life. Buruli ulcer maims, especially when limbs have to be amputated to save a life. Human African trypanosomiasis (sleeping sickness) severely debilitates before it kills, and mortality approaches 100% in untreated cases. Without post-exposure prophylaxis, rabies causes acute encephalitis and is always fatal. Leishmaniasis, in its various forms, leaves deep and permanent scars or entirely destroys the mucous membranes of the nose, mouth and throat. In its most severe form, it attacks the internal organs and is rapidly fatal if untreated. Chagas disease can cause young adults to develop heart conditions, so that they fill hospital beds instead of the labour force. Severe schistosomiasis disrupts school attendance, contributes to malnutrition and impairs the cognitive development of children. Guinea-worm disease causes excruciating, debilitating pain, sometimes for extended periods and often coinciding with the peak agricultural season. Dengue has emerged as a rapidly spreading vector-borne disease affecting mostly poor, urban populations; it is also the leading cause of hospital admissions in several countries.

The consequences are costly for societies and for health care. Such costs include intensive care for dengue haemorrhagic fever and clinical rabies, surgery and prolonged hospital stays for Chagas disease and Buruli ulcer, and rehabilitation for leprosy and lymphatic filariasis. For some diseases, such as sleeping sickness and leishmaniasis, treatments are old, cumbersome to administer and toxic. For others, especially the diseases that cause blindness, the damage is permanent. Clinical development of rabies can be prevented through timely immunization after exposure, but access to life-saving biologicals is expensive and is not affordable in many Asian and African countries. For most of these diseases, stigma and social exclusion compound the misery, especially for women.

Fortunately, these problems are now much better documented and much more widely recognized. They are also being addressed. Recent developments on several fronts have radically changed the prospects for controlling these diseases, and new initiatives are enabling the people left behind by socioeconomic progress to catch up. The ambitions for health development have broadened, creating space for neglected tropical diseases. The Millennium Declaration and its Goals recognize the contribution of health to the overarching objective of reducing poverty. Efforts to control neglected tropical diseases constitute a pro-poor strategy on a grand scale. The logic has changed: instead of waiting for these diseases to gradually disappear as countries develop and living conditions improve, a deliberate effort to make them disappear is now viewed as a route to poverty alleviation that can itself spur socioeconomic development.

As this report shows, reaching such an objective is now entirely feasible for the masses of people known to be affected or at risk. Good medicines are available for many of these diseases, and research continues to document their safety and efficacy when administered individually or in combination. Generous drug donations by pharmaceutical companies have helped relieve some of the financial barriers and allowed programmes to scale up coverage. A strategy of preventive chemotherapy, which mimics the advantages of childhood immunization, is being used to protect entire at-risk populations and reduce the reservoir of infection. The fact that many of these diseases overlap geographically has practical advantages: preventive chemotherapy regimens are being integrated so that several diseases can be tackled together, thus streamlining operational demands and cutting costs. An integrated approach to vector management likewise maximizes the use of resources and tools for controlling vector-borne diseases.

Governments and foundations have contributed substantial funds. Research to develop new tools (such as medicines, diagnostics, vaccines and medical devices) and improve the delivery of existing ones has increased. The momentum continues to grow. As the report shows, nearly 670 million people had been reached with preventive chemotherapy by the end of 2008. For some of these diseases, evidence indicates that, when a certain threshold of population coverage is reached, transmission drops significantly; this raises the possibility that several of these ancient diseases could be eliminated by 2020 if current efforts to scale up interventions for preventive chemotherapy are increased.

While the report highlights a number of remaining challenges, the overall message is overwhelmingly positive. It is entirely possible to control neglected tropical diseases. Aiming at their complete control and even elimination is fully justified, and this report sets out the solid evidence needed to achieve control. Above all, it makes the case for doing more, as an international community, to relieve hidden misery, on a grand scale, among people who would otherwise suffer in silence.

Dr Margaret Chan
Director-General
World Health Organization

Executive summary

Neglected tropical diseases (NTDs) blight the lives of a billion people worldwide and threaten the health of millions more. These ancient companions of poverty weaken impoverished populations, frustrate the achievement of health in the Millennium Development Goals and impede global development outcomes. A more reliable evaluation of their significance to public health and economies has convinced governments, donors, the pharmaceutical industry and other agencies, including nongovernmental organizations (NGOs), to invest in preventing and controlling this diverse group of diseases. Global efforts to control "hidden" diseases, such as dracunculiasis (guinea-worm disease), leprosy, schistosomiasis, lymphatic filariasis and yaws, have yielded progressive health gains including the imminent eradication of dracunculiasis. Since 1989 (when most endemic countries began reporting monthly from each endemic village), the number of new dracunculiasis cases has fallen from 892 055 in 12 endemic countries to 3190 in 4 countries in 2009, a decrease of more than 99%.

The World Health Organization (WHO) recommends five public-health strategies for the prevention and control of NTDs: preventive chemotherapy; intensified case-management; vector control; the provision of safe water, sanitation and hygiene; and veterinary public health (that is, applying veterinary sciences to ensure the health and well-being of humans). Although one approach may predominate for control of a specific disease or group of diseases, evidence suggests that more effective control results when all five approaches are combined and delivered locally.

Activities to prevent and control NTDs are included in the policies and budgets of many endemic countries. This has led to the development of interventions that are appropriate to existing health systems, often with the support of implementing partners. Overall, at least 670 million people in 75 countries benefitted from preventive chemotherapy during 2008, although not all were given the full package of medicines. Lymphatic filariasis, onchocerciasis, schistosomiasis, soil-transmitted helminthiases and trachoma are being controlled mostly through this approach. These are a group of infections with a high disease burden for which safe and simple treatments are available.

Actions to address the suffering caused by NTDs and assess how their impact extends into sectors other than health will promote development by breaking the cycle of poverty and disease; foster health security by reducing the vulnerability of human and animal populations to infection; and strengthen health systems by embedding strategic approaches and locally appropriate interventions into national health programmes. The development of regional plans in response to the *Global plan to combat neglected tropical diseases 2008–2015* has also led to growing awareness of NTDs and the suffering they cause.

The involvement of the pharmaceutical industry in NTDs, and subsequent donations made to support their control, have increased access to high-quality medicines free of charge for hundreds of millions of poor people. The increasing willingness and commitment of local and global communities of partners to work with endemic countries have brought resources, innovation, expertise and advocacy to efforts to overcome NTDs. Intersectoral collaboration, involving education, nutrition and agriculture, has reinforced NTD control.

Achieving and sustaining intensified control of NTDs will be a critical milestone for WHO in realizing its objective that all people attain the highest possible level of health. For example, the number of notified new cases of the chronic form of human African trypanosomiasis (*T. b. gambiense*) has fallen by 62%, from 27 862 in 1999 to 10 372 in 2008, and the number of newly reported cases of the acute form (*T. b. rhodesiense*) has fallen by 58%, from 619 to 259, due largely to intensified case-detection and management.

This report also identifies challenges that will have to be faced if the current achievements in NTD prevention and control are to be sustained and extended. Despite global economic constraints, support from Spain, the United Kingdom, the United States, other countries, agencies and NGOs will need to be sustained. These commitments should encourage others to expand their support for developing the services needed to overcome NTDs.

Planning for the development and control of NTDs should take into account the effects of porous borders, population growth and migration, urbanization, the movement of livestock and vectors, and the political and geographical consequences of climate change. Several of these factors help to explain the rapidly increasing global spread of dengue. From 2001 to 2009, a total of 6 626 950 cases were reported to WHO from more than 30 countries in WHO's Region of the Americas, where all four serotypes of the virus circulate. During the same period, there were 180 216 cases of dengue haemorrhagic fever and 2498 deaths reported to WHO. Dengue has resurged in the region because successful vector surveillance and control measures were not sustained after the campaign to eradicate *Aedes aegypti*, the principal vector, during the 1960s and early 1970s. Explosive outbreaks now occur every 3–5 years. The South-East Asia Region accounts for most deaths, but the decline in case-fatality rates since 2007 has been attributed mainly to effective training in standardized case-management, based on a network of expertise, and training materials developed by Member countries in the region.

As control interventions reach more people and new technology is embraced, quicker responses will need to be made to information about the epidemiology, transmission and burden of NTDs. Similarly, programme managers will need to react quickly to information about the coverage, compliance, acceptance and impact of interventions.

Expertise in individual NTDs is lacking in some countries and continues to decline in others. The decline in expertise is severe in the areas of vector control, case-management, pesticide management and veterinary aspects of public health. The ways to prevent and control rabies – a zoonotic disease that kills tens of thousands of people annually in Africa and Asia and necessitates post-exposure prophylaxis of more than 14 million patients worldwide following contact with suspect rabid animals – are not known or well understood in many countries where the disease exists.

As expansion of prevention and control activities increases, the need to strengthen health systems, and to train and support staff in technical and management expertise, will become more urgent.

Targets for coverage set by the World Health Assembly for control of lymphatic filariasis, schistosomiasis, soil-transmitted helminthiases and trachoma will not be met, especially in WHO's African and South-East Asia regions, unless interventions with preventive chemotherapy increase. In 2008, only 8% of people with schistosomiasis had access to high-quality medicines. Donations of praziquantel from the private sector, and funds for its production, are insufficient to provide the quantities of this essential medicine needed to control schistosomiasis. The provision of medicines to treat soil-transmitted helminthiases also must be increased significantly. Production of medicines used to treat NTDs must be made more attractive to companies that manufacture generic pharmaceuticals.

A research strategy is required to develop and implement new medicines, notably for leishmaniasis and trypanosomiasis; new methods for vector control; vaccines for dengue; and new diagnostics that will be accessible to all who need them.

The Strategic Technical and Advisory Group for NTDs, at its meeting in Geneva in late June 2010, reviewed this report and commended it to the community dedicated to the global prevention and control of these diseases of poverty.

The theme at the global partners' meeting in Geneva in April 2007 was that a turning point had been reached in the efforts to overcome NTDs. The content of this report demonstrates that there can be no turning back: the concept of "neglected" is confined to the history of public health.

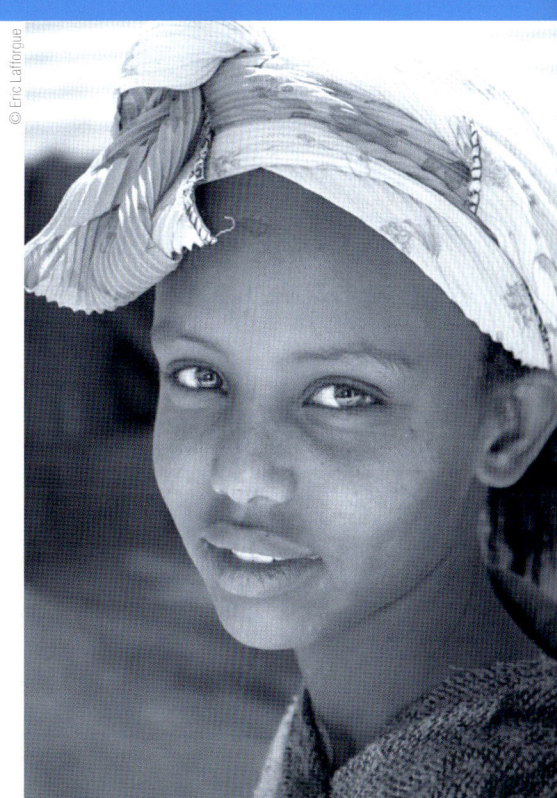

1 Neglected tropical diseases: a paradigm shift

In 2003, the World Health Organization (WHO) initiated a paradigm shift in the control and elimination of a group of neglected tropical diseases (NTDs). The process – led by the former Director-General, the late Dr JW Lee – involved an important strategic change, from a traditional approach centred on diseases to one responding to the health needs of marginalized communities.

The new approach uses integrated interventions based on tools for controlling NTDs. From a public-health perspective, this change translated into the provision of care and the delivery of treatment to underserved populations. The shift ensures a more efficient use of limited resources and the alleviation of poverty and accompanying illness for millions of people living in rural and urban areas.

This emerging vision was sharpened at a meeting held in Berlin, Germany, in December 2003 that convened experts from diverse sectors, including public health, economics, human rights, research, nongovernmental organizations (NGOs) and the pharmaceutical industry. The meeting set the scene for WHO to translate the new approach into a strategic policy and formulate ways of providing poor populations with an effective and comprehensive solution to some of their health problems. From 2003 to 2007, bold steps were taken to develop a framework for tackling NTDs in a coordinated and integrated way. Details of the framework are set out in section 4 of this report and in WHO's *Global plan to combat neglected tropical diseases 2008–2015*.

1.1 Common features of neglected tropical diseases

The 17 neglected tropical diseases profiled in this report share several common features, which are summarized in *Box 1.4.1*. The most profound commonality is their stranglehold on populations whose lives are ravaged by poverty. During the past decade, the international community's recognition of this unacceptable situation has stimulated the growth of a community of partners committed to resolving this double bind of disease and poverty. Working to overcome the impact of NTDs represents a largely untapped development opportunity to alleviate the poverty of many populations and thereby make a direct impact on the achievement of the Millennium Development Goals (MDGs) as well as fulfilling WHO's mission: ensuring attainment of the highest standard of health as a fundamental human right of all peoples.

1.2 New strategic approaches

Preventive chemotherapy – a strategy first used for delivering anthelminthic medicines by means of a population-based approach – focuses on optimizing the use of single-administration medicines targeted simultaneously at more than one form of helminthiasis. Efforts to tackle helminth infections in a coordinated fashion can be traced back to the 2001 World Health Assembly resolution WHA54.19 on schistosomiasis and soil-transmitted helminth infections, which set common objectives and goals for their prevention and control.

Five years later in 2006, this concept was further developed when WHO published a manual on preventive chemotherapy in human helminthiases recommending the integrated implementation of disease interventions against the four main helminth infections (lymphatic filariasis, onchocerciasis, schistosomiasis and soil-transmitted helminthiases) based on the coordinated use of a set of powerful anthelminthic medicines with an impressive safety record. Preventive chemotherapy is now implemented worldwide and is used to treat more than half a billion people every year.

The success of preventive chemotherapy is attributable to a number of factors including:

> the impact of preventive chemotherapy in reducing morbidity and sustaining decreases in transmission;
>
> demonstration of the association of helminth infections with poverty and disadvantage, and of the geographical overlap of the four main helminth infections targeted;
>
> the added benefit of controlling a number of infections and infestations not specifically targeted by the intervention (such as strongyloidiasis, scabies and lice);

flexibility of treatment that allows the expansion of its target to other helminth infections (such as fascioliasis and other foodborne trematode infections).

The use of existing mechanisms to deliver anthelminthic medicines provides a platform to target other communicable diseases (such as trachoma) and paves the way for expansion of a public-health approach that shares common features with immunization.

For protozoan and bacterial diseases, such as human African trypanosomiasis (sleeping sickness), leishmaniasis, Chagas disease and Buruli ulcer (*Mycobacterium ulcerans* infection), the new focus on improved and timely access to specialized care through improved case detection and decentralized clinical management is intended to prevent mortality, reduce morbidity and interrupt transmission.

Tackling these diseases effectively requires specific and profound expertise. In the long term, WHO must ensure that sustainable steps are being taken to prevent these diseases and to promote the development of better, safer, more affordable and simpler-to-use diagnostic methods and medicines.

Until such methods become available, the focus remains on optimizing the use of existing treatments and expanding their access to a greater number of people, who may immediately benefit from a more coordinated strategic approach, through innovative and intensified case-management.

The approach to vector control has also been revisited in light of the new, integrated strategic framework. Vector control now serves as an important cross-cutting activity aimed at enhancing the impact and the performance of both preventive chemotherapy and case-management. Integrated vector management is an effective combination of different interventions and forms part of an intersectoral and interprogrammatic collaboration within the health sector and with other sectors, including agriculture and the environment. Its aim is to improve the efficacy, cost-effectiveness, ecological soundness and sustainability of disease control implemented against vector-borne NTDs.

1.3 Refocusing

Following its second meeting in Berlin in 2005, WHO proposed that the vaguely defined term "other communicable diseases" be changed to the more sharply focused "neglected tropical diseases". This change neatly encapsulated the paradigm shift responsible for the new approach to dealing with NTDs. The change recognizes that NTD control can be achieved if three requirements are met: (i) attention and action are given to the needs of populations affected by

NTDs rather than to their diseases; (ii) interventions to deliver treatments are integrated with control measures; and (iii) evidence-based advocacy is deployed to generate resources for control from the international community.

In April 2007, WHO convened its first meeting of Global Partners on NTDs, which was attended by more than 200 participants, including representatives from WHO's Member States, United Nations agencies, the World Bank, philanthropic foundations, universities, pharmaceutical companies, international NGOs and other institutions dedicated to contributing their time, efforts and resources to tackling these diseases.

1.4 Lessons learnt

The paradigm shift has enabled Member States and partners to find innovative solutions to enable weak health systems to target the people most in need: the poorest sectors of the population with limited or non-existent financial means.

Grouping several diseases together under a new conceptual framework presents an opportunity to recalculate the collective burden associated with this set of diverse afflictions as well as their cumulative public-health relevance. The framework has also enabled WHO to raise the profile of NTDs and to mobilize resources for scaling up implementation of activities for their global control and elimination.

This report is confined to 17 NTDs, although some comprise separate infections and thus separate diseases: for example, soil-transmitted helminthiases comprise three separate infections and therefore three separate diseases. There are 149 countries and territories where NTDs are endemic, at least 100 of which are endemic for 2 or more diseases, and 30 countries that are endemic for 6 or more.

Box 1.4.1 Common features of neglected tropical diseases

A proxy for poverty and disadvantage

Neglected tropical diseases have an enormous impact on individuals, families and communities in developing countries in terms of disease burden, quality of life, loss of productivity and the aggravation of poverty as well as the high cost of long-term care. They constitute a serious obstacle to socioeconomic development and quality of life at all levels.

Affect populations with low visibility and little political voice

This group of diseases largely affects low-income and politically marginalized people living in rural and urban areas. Such people cannot readily influence administrative and governmental decisions that affect their health, and often seem to have no constituency that speaks on their behalf. Diseases associated with rural poverty may have little impact on decision-makers in capital cities and their expanding populations.

Do not travel widely

Unlike influenza, HIV/AIDS and malaria and, to a lesser extent, tuberculosis, most NTDs generally do not spread widely, and so present little threat to the inhabitants of high-income countries. Rather, their distribution is restricted by climate and its effect on the distribution of vectors and reservoir hosts; in most cases, there appears to be a low risk of transmission beyond the tropics.

Cause stigma and discrimination, especially of girls and women

Many NTDs cause disfigurement and disability, leading to stigma and social discrimination. In some cases, their impact disproportionately affects girls and women, whose marriage prospects may diminish or who may be left vulnerable to abuse and abandonment. Some NTDs contribute to adverse pregnancy outcomes.

Have an important impact on morbidity and mortality

The once-widespread assumptions held by the international community that people at risk of NTDs experience relatively little morbidity, and that these diseases have low rates of mortality, have been comprehensively refuted. A large body of evidence, published in peer-reviewed medical and scientific journals, has demonstrated the nature and extent of the adverse effects of NTDs.

Are relatively neglected by research

Research is needed to develop new diagnostics and medicines, and to make accessible interventions to prevent, cure and manage the complications of all NTDs.

Can be controlled, prevented and possibly eliminated using effective and feasible solutions

The five strategic interventions recommended by WHO (preventive chemotherapy; intensified case-management; vector control; the provision of safe water, sanitation and hygiene; and veterinary public health) make feasible control, prevention and even elimination of several NTDs. Costs are relatively low.

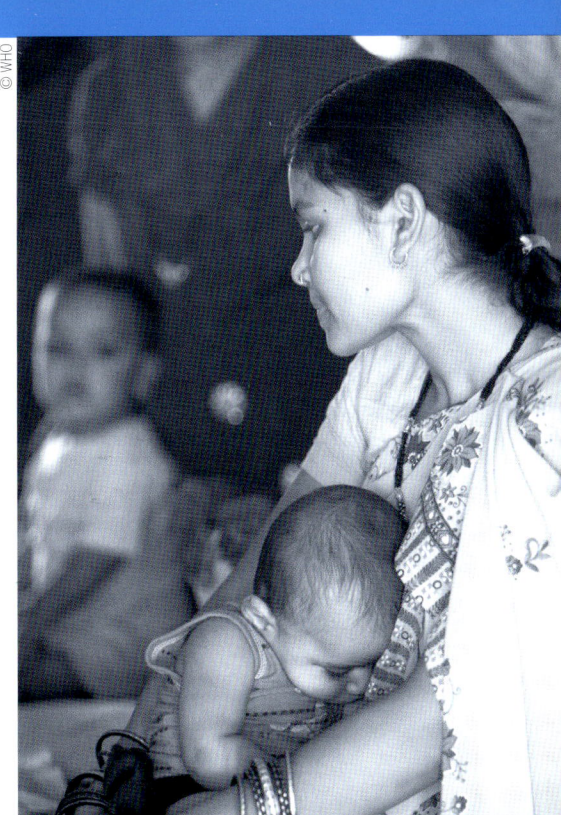

2 Sixty years of growing concern

Since its founding in 1948, WHO has led the common endeavour of protecting people from infectious diseases, recognizing that the interests of its Member States are best served if the peoples of other countries are also helped to live in healthy conditions (*1*).

This report is the first of its kind to review WHO's work to prevent, control, eliminate and eradicate 17 NTDs. Section 5 provides a detailed account of these diseases. History shows that NTDs have not been overlooked or neglected by WHO (*2*). The Fifth World Health Assembly, held in Geneva, Switzerland, in May 1952, addressed the technical assistance needed by countries to deal with treponematoses, rabies, leprosy, trachoma, hookworm, schistosomiasis and both forms of filariasis (*3*). These diseases are included in WHO's mandate today (*4, 5*), and it remains committed and available to attend to requests for prevention and control from countries where NTDs are endemic.

In some ways, application of the term "neglected" to the communicable diseases discussed in this report may appear inappropriate, since it is clear that WHO has never neglected them. Rather, WHO has consistently highlighted the impact that these diseases impose on its Member States. The overt consequences of infection with the causative agents of NTDs include skin ulcers, blindness, limb deformities and chronic pain. Less evident, but no less debilitating, are lesions to internal organs, anaemia, growth retardation, impairment of cognitive development, exercise intolerance and fatigue, and the impairment of mental functions through neurological sequelae. These conditions blight the social, educational and professional lives of populations affected by NTDS, most of whom are poor people. Left untreated, diseases such as dengue haemorrhagic fever, human African trypanosomiasis, visceral leishmaniasis and rabies are commonly fatal.

The heavy burden imposed by NTDs on poor people has been gaining wider recognition and prominence in countries and by institutions with the capacity to release resources for prevention and control. Effective advocacy has successfully exploited the notion of "neglected" and stimulated health policy-makers to work to overcome NTDs in harmony with the ideals and aims of the MDGs. Tools for treatment interventions in communities can now reach the millions in need.

Resources are needed to support the research required to develop new medicines and diagnostics, to produce and test tools for interventions, and to facilitate the clinical management of several NTDs.

Advocacy to support activities to overcome NTDs must continue if resources for extending sustainable relief are to be forthcoming. A record of the scale of the most encouraging global response has been published in the *Report of the global partners' meeting on neglected tropical diseases* (6). In effect, partners at that meeting demonstrated their response to "the Golden Rule", displayed as a mosaic by the 20th-century American painter and illustrator Norman Rockwell on a wall in the headquarters of the United Nations in New York: "Do unto others as you would have them do unto you".

2.1 World Health Assembly resolutions

Every year, the World Health Assembly – the supreme decision-making body of WHO – evaluates the status of different health problems and decides whether the adoption of a specific resolution will add impetus to the effort designed to bring relief, and so improve the quality of life of populations at risk. The first resolution on what are now termed NTDs was adopted by the Second World Health Assembly in 1949 (*Annex 1*).

2.2 Landmarks in prevention and control

In addition to the work underpinning and justifying the resolutions of the World Health Assembly, a series of initiatives has been proposed to form partnerships, strengthen measures and raise financial and other support to prevent and control NTDs (*Table 2.2.1*).

Table 2.2.1 Summary of landmarks in overcoming neglected tropical diseases

Year	Event
1948	World Health Organization (WHO) begins work
	WHO establishes Veterinary Public Health Programme
1952	UNICEF and WHO launch Global Yaws Programme
1960	WHO launches Programme for the Evaluation and Testing of New Insecticides
1974	Onchocerciasis Control Programme for West Africa begins
1976	Special Programme for Research and Training in Tropical Diseases established
1982	The Carter Center is inaugurated and begins work
1987	Mectizan® Donation Program created
1995	International Commission for the Certification of Dracunculiasis Eradication established
	African Programme for Onchocerciasis Control set up
1997	Programme Against African Trypanosomiasis established
	WHO-GET 2020 Alliance (Global Elimination of Trachoma by the year 2020) created
1998	Prime Minister Hashimoto of Japan presents his parasite-control initiative to the G8 Meeting
	Global Buruli Ulcer Initiative established
	Médecins Sans Frontières initiates a fund to fight neglected tropical diseases from the proceeds of its Nobel Peace Prize
1999	WHO Study Group on Future Trends in Veterinary Public Health established
2000	WHO Global Programme to Eliminate Lymphatic Filariasis launched
	Bill & Melinda Gates Foundation created
	Pan African Tsetse and Trypanosomiasis Eradication Campaign created
2002	WHO publishes *Global defence against the infectious disease threat*
	Publication of the first version of the *WHO model formulary*
2003	First issue of WHO's newsletter *Action Against Worms*
	Drugs for Neglected Diseases Initiative established
	Berlin, Germany, hosts workshop on intensified control of neglected diseases
2004	Third global meeting of the Partners for Parasite Control, leading to publication of *Deworming for health and development*
2005	Strategic and technical meeting on intensified control of neglected tropical diseases held in Berlin, Germany
	First International Conference on the Control of Neglected Zoonotic Diseases: a route to poverty alleviation held at WHO headquarters in Geneva, Switzerland
	WHO Department of Control of Neglected Tropical Diseases established
	Bangladesh, India and Nepal sign an agreement to eliminate visceral leishmaniasis by 2015
2006	Collaboration begins between WHO and the Foundation for Innovative New Diagnostics to develop and evaluate new diagnostic tests for human African trypanosomiasis
	Preventive chemotherapy in human helminthiasis: coordinated use of anthelminthic drugs in control interventions. A manual for health professionals and programme managers published by WHO
2007	Global partners' meeting on neglected tropical diseases held at WHO headquarters in Geneva, Switzerland
	Joint meeting on Integrated Control of Neglected Zoonotic Diseases in Africa, held in Nairobi, Kenya
2008	Launch of the Neglected Tropical Disease Initiative by the Government of the United States
	Announcement that neglected tropical diseases are to be targeted following a new £50 million commitment from the Department for International Development of the Government of the United Kingdom

Most important has been the development by WHO of a framework for action that gives equal attention to neglected communities and their health problems. The communities where NTDs are entrenched have limited financial resources, a shortage of trained health workers and an urgent need for a stronger infrastructure to facilitate the delivery of health services (7). Implementation of this framework still depends heavily on input from countries where NTDs are not endemic. The response has been significant, thanks to bilateral donations, the generosity of the pharmaceutical industry, and the work of NGOs, implementing agencies, universities and philanthropic institutions.

There is, however, growing recognition that successful and sustainable control depend on the political commitment and ownership of interventions by governments of countries where the diseases are endemic. In his Annual Report of 1951 (8), Dr Brock Chisholm – the first Director-General of WHO – was aware of this essential aspect of NTD control. He declared, "Too often countries requesting assistance have been the object of well-meaning but disastrous attempts to superimpose on the local culture foreign patterns which, lacking the necessary foundations, are bound to result in friction, misunderstanding and ultimate failure. In health work, as in all other fields of technical assistance, there can be no question of simply transplanting techniques from one place to another".

2.3 Strategic and Technical Advisory Group for Neglected Tropical Diseases

In 2007, WHO established a Strategic and Technical Advisory Group for neglected tropical diseases to support actions taken to overcome these diseases. The group serves as the principal advisory group to WHO and the Director-General on matters relating to the prevention and control of NTDs worldwide. Its main objective is to support the achievement of the goals contained in the *Global plan to combat neglected tropical diseases 2008–2015* (5). Members have expertise in the range of NTDs and represent disease-endemic countries, academia, donors and agencies; the group is supported by WHO's regional staff and secretariat.

In response to advice from the Strategic and Technical Advisory Group, and after consultation with the global NTD community, WHO established three working groups, each with a remit to cover key aspects of managing the control of NTDs:

> Working Group on access to quality-assured, essential medicines for NTD control, concerned with improving implementation, increasing effectiveness, using economies of scale and developing faster self-reliance by health authorities in endemic countries.

Working Group on monitoring and evaluation, concerned with the needs of national programmes, monitoring disease-specific indicators, and monitoring coverage of interventions and their impact.

Working Group on anthelminthic drug efficacy, concerned with the possible emergence of drug resistance, which could accelerate as access to preventive chemotherapy expands.

REFERENCES

1. Brockington F. *World health*. Harmondsworth, Penguin Books Ltd., 1958.
2. Account of the First World Health Assembly. *Chronicle of the World Health Organization*, 1948, 177(2):180–182.
3. Account of the Fifth World Health Assembly. *Chronicle of the World Health Organization*, 1952, 6:161–250.
4. *Global defence against the infectious disease threat*. Geneva, World Health Organization, 2003 (WHO/CDS/2003.15).
5. *Global plan to combat neglected tropical diseases 2008–2015*. Geneva, World Health Organization, 2007 (WHO/CDS/NTD/2007.3).
6. *Report of the global partners' meeting on neglected tropical diseases: a turning point*. Geneva, World Health Organization, 2007 (WHO/CDS/NTD/2007.4).
7. *Intensified control of neglected diseases: report of an international workshop, Berlin, 10–12 December 2003*. Geneva, World Health Organization, 2004 (WHO/CDS/CPE/CEE/2004.45).
8. The work WHO: 1951. Annual report of the Director-General to the World Health Assembly and to the United Nations. *Chronicle of the World Health Organization*, 1952, 6(7-8):170.

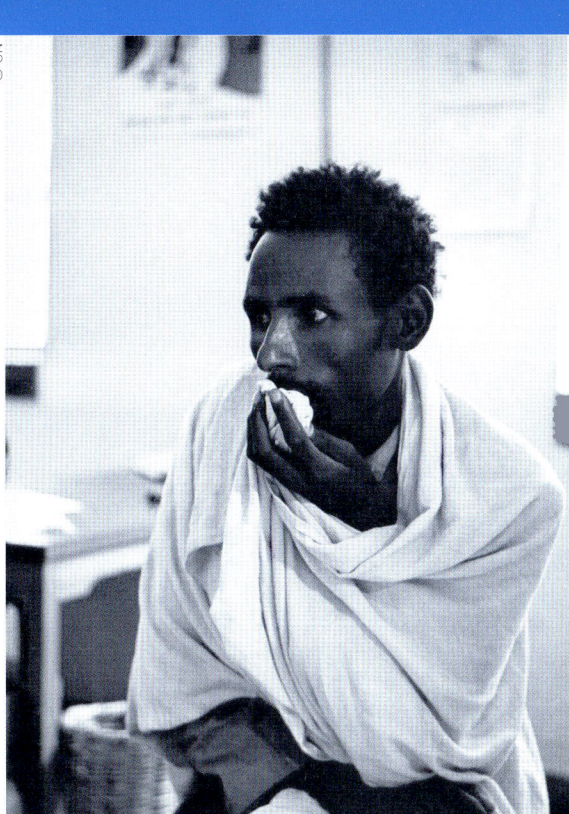

3 Human and economic burden

P ublic-health planners face the problem of setting priorities for attention – a necessary task since competition for the most effective use of resources is inevitable.

3.1 Epidemiological burden

The concept of DALYs (disability-adjusted life years) was developed to enable the burden of individual diseases to be assessed quantitatively and comparatively. The number of DALYs assigned to a specific disease at a particular time gives an estimate of the sum of years of potential life lost due to premature mortality and the years of productive life lost. WHO's Department of Health Statistics and Informatics has compiled and published estimates of DALYs for 2004 (*1*). The DALYs for a selection of NTDs discussed in this report are set out in *Table 3.1.1*.

Table 3.1.1 Estimated number of disability-adjusted life years (DALYs) (in thousands) by cause (neglected tropical disease), and by WHO region (excluding the European Region)[a], 2004

Neglected tropical disease	World[b]	WHO region				
		African	Americas	Eastern Mediterranean	South-East Asia	Western Pacific
Human African trypanosomiasis	1 673	1 609	0	62	0	0
Chagas disease	430	0	426	0	0	0
Schistosomiasis	1 707	1 502	46	145	0	13
Leishmaniasis	1 974	328	45	281	1 264	51
Lymphatic filariasis	5 941	2 263	10	75	3 525	65
Onchocerciasis	389	375	1	11	0	0
Leprosy	194	25	16	22	118	13
Dengue	670	9	73	28	391	169
Trachoma	1 334	601	15	208	88	419
Ascariasis[c]	1 851	915	60	162	404	308
Trichuriasis[c]	1 012	236	73	61	372	269
Hookworm disease[c]	1 092	377	20	43	286	364

[a] Source: *The global burden of disease: 2004 update* (*1*).
[b] Because estimates from the European Region were omitted from the table, numbers for the regions may not always add up to the world's total.
[c] Soil-transmitted helminthiases.
 The published sources from which these tables are based should be consulted for details of the costs involved.

There is consensus about the need for DALYs or an objective measure of the burden of disease. However, there is some criticism of the procedures used to make the estimates, and considerable concern about the quality and reliability of the raw data available for generating the estimates. Four reasons may be offered to support this cause for concern. Firstly, for any disease there may be little information on numbers of cases and deaths because surveillance systems and platforms for most NTDs and infections in animal reservoirs are weak or non-existent. Secondly, national and regional estimates for some diseases are often derived from a few studies carried out in high-risk populations. Thirdly, for some conditions, such as schistosomiasis, there is uncertainty about the accuracy of the disability weights that should be attached to small or moderate reductions in physical function, to pain and to other forms of impairment. Small differences in disability weights, when multiplied by large numbers of affected people, yield highly variable estimates of DALYs lost. Fourthly, the less overt or subtle morbidity of the highly prevalent NTDs affects the severity of concurrent infection and disease. DALY estimates still have to take account of this complication.

Estimates of DALYs for Buruli ulcer, cysticercosis, dracunculiasis, echinococcosis, endemic syphilis, foodborne trematode infections (clonorchiasis, fascioliasis, opisthorchiasis) and rabies are not explicitly stated. However, they contribute to the burden of disease caused by NTDs, and some have exceedingly high mortality if left undiagnosed and untreated.

3.2 Economic burden

Data about the economic burden of NTDs are confined to small studies in limited geographical areas. More work is needed to quantify the impact of NTDs on the productivity of women. Where data exist, the economic impact is significant. For example, lymphatic filariasis causes almost US$ 1 billion a year in lost productivity (*2*) and the annual global expenditure for rabies prevention and control exceeds US$ 1 billion, by WHO's conservative assessment.

3.2.1 Economic impact

There is an unquantifiable dimension to the burden of NTDs that saps the unpaid work and productivity of millions of women. In countries where NTDs are endemic, women are the caregivers when children and family members are healthy and when they are sick; they collect water and fuel, grow vegetables and tend crops, provide meals and maintain the household (*3*). This vital work is unpaid and would be easier if women were relieved from the burden of NTDs. In low-income countries, children are an economic resource, and improving their health will help them better perform their daily tasks.

A quantifiable dimension to the burden of disease caused by NTDs is the loss of productivity and its impact on the productivity of individuals, households, communities and nations. That people with poor health and crippling disabilities are less productive than their healthy counterparts cannot be challenged, but carefully stratified analyses of the results of well-designed, large-scale investigations are rare. Understanding the effect of NTDs on productivity will help promote prevention and control activities, and assure governments and donors that resources directed towards these endeavours are a good investment. Information about the impact of several NTDs is shown in *Table 3.2.1.1.*

Table 3.2.1.1 Economic costs of selected neglected tropical diseases[a] (data are the latest available)

Disease	Setting	Reported productivity loss[b]
Chagas disease	Latin America	Estimated 752 000 working days/year lost due to premature deaths. US$ 1.2 billion/year in lost productivity in 7 southernmost countries. Absenteeism of workers affected by Chagas disease in Brazil represented an estimated minimum loss of US$ 5.6 million/year.[c]
Cysticercosis	Eastern Cape province (South Africa), Honduras, India	The societal monetary cost of *Taenia solium* cysticercosis was estimated at US$ 15.27 million (95% CI US$ 51.6–299 million) in India, US$ 28.3 million (US$ 7.1–42.9 million) in Honduras and US$ 16.6 million (US$ 8.3–22.8 million) in the Eastern Cape province (South Africa). The total annual costs associated with cysticercosis were estimated at US$ 13 million; the monetary burden per case of human cysticercosis amounted to US$ 252.
Dengue fever	India	The average total economic burden was estimated at US$ 29.3 million (US$ 27.5–31.1 million). Costs in the private health sector were estimated to be almost 4 times that of public sector expenditures.
Echinococcosis	Global	The financial burden of the disease in estimates of purchasing power parity is 4.1 billion international dollars annually, of which 46% is due to human treatment and morbidity and 54% is associated animal-health costs.
Lymphatic filariasis	Various countries	Annual economic burden of lymphatic filariasis measured in lost productivity reported in 1998 was about US$ 1.7 billion in 2008, taking into account inflation in countries that are part of the African Programme for Onchocerciasis Control. ERRs are 25% at the end of the investment period in 2019, and 28% over 30 years. The programme breaks even in the tenth year. Lymphatic filariasis causes almost US$ 1.3 billion/year in lost productivity.
Soil-transmitted helminthiases	Kenya	On the basis of the estimated rate of return to education in Kenya, deworming is likely to increase the net present value of wages by more than US$ 40 per treated person. Benefit-to-cost ratio = 100. Deworming may increase adult income by 40%.
Schistosomiasis	Philippines	After a series of computations, of which the disability rate was regarded as the most important, a total of 45.4 days off-work lost per infected person/year was obtained.
Trachoma	Various countries	The economic cost of trachoma in terms of lost productivity is estimated at US$ 2.9 billion annually.

CI = confidence interval; ERR = economic rate of return.
[a] Source: Reproduced with permission from Conteh L et al. (*4*).
[b] All costs and losses are inflated from their original year of calculation and converted to their 2008 US$ equivalent with a constant dollar rate.
[c] The base year of costs is not given, so costs remain in original form.
The published sources from which these tables are based should be consulted for details of the costs involved.

3.2.2 Costs of interventions

Assessing the burden of NTDs in terms of DALYs is a powerful approach that can be used to evaluate the gains made, and the costs of interventions for their prevention and control. Put simply, how many DALYs can be averted by investing fully in a programme to control NTDs (including the costs of planning, administration, staffing, training, community relations, logistics, medicines, procurement and reporting)? For example, the cost of treating a patient with lymphatic filariasis using ivermectin and albendazole (donated by Merck & Co., Inc., and GlaxoSmithKline) ranges from US$ 0.05 to US$ 0.10 per person treated, while the cost of the DALYs averted is reckoned to be US$ 5.90. Results of this sort are encouraging for NTD control provided that the full costs of intervention have been identified.

An economic analysis of deworming campaigns among school-aged children conducted in seven countries (Cambodia, Egypt, Ghana, the Lao People's Democratic Republic, Myanmar, the United Republic of Tanzania and Viet Nam) calculated a cost of US$ 0.07 per each round of drug distribution (or US$ 70 000 to cover 1 million school-aged children), with minimal variation among countries (*5*). This calculation includes the costs of training, health education, procurement and distribution of medicines, media campaigns, monitoring and supervision.

Economic evaluations of the Onchocerciasis Control Programme in west Africa show a net present value (equivalent discounted benefits minus discounted costs) of US$ 919 million for the programme over 39 years, using a conservative 10% rate to discount future health and productivity gains. The net present value for the African Programme for Onchocerciasis Control is calculated at US$ 121 million over 21 years, also using a 10% discount rate. However, the economic success of ivermectin distribution is sensitive to the fact that the drug itself has been donated. The market value of donations made by Merck & Co. Inc., to the African Programme for Onchocerciasis Control for just 1 year considerably outweighs the benefits calculated for both the Onchocerciasis Control Programme and the African Programme for Onchocerciasis Control over the duration of these projects.

Table 3.2.2.1 summarizes the findings of an attempt to calculate the DALYs averted for several NTDs in relation to the costs of their treatment and control. The published sources from which this table is based should be consulted for details of the costs involved.

Table 3.2.2.1 Cost-effectiveness of controlling neglected tropical diseases[a]

Disease	Intervention	Cost per DALY averted (US$)
Chagas disease	Vector control	317
Lymphatic filariasis	In implementation units (districts) where prevalence is greater than 1%, annual mass drug administration to treat the entire at-risk population for 5–7 years: ivermectin and albendazole in Africa, and diethylcarbamazine and albendazole in onchocerciasis-free countries:	5–10
	• to interrupt transmission and achieve elimination of the public-health problem	35
	• to initiate morbidity control, surgery and lymphoedema management	1–4
	To provide salt fortified with diethylcarbamazine (China)	59–370
	Vector control	
Schistosomiasis	Mass school-based treatment with praziquantel and albendazole combined with schistosomiasis treatment	10–23
	Mass school-based treatment with praziquantel alone	410–844
Trachoma	Trachoma control based on SAFE strategy (Surgery, Antibiotic treatment, Face washing and Environmental control)	5–100
Onchocerciasis	Community-directed treatment programmes with ivermectin	9
Soil-transmitted helminthiases (hookworm, roundworm, and whipworm)	Mass school-based treatment with albendazole or mebendazole	2–11
Leprosy	Case-detection and treatment with multidrug therapy using donated drugs	46
	Prevention of disability	1–122
Dengue fever control	Case-management	716–1757
	Environmental control	more than 2440
Leishmaniasis	Case detection and treatment; vector control.	11–22
Human African trypanosomiasis	Case-finding and treatment:	
	• with melarsoprol	Less than 12
	• with eflornithine	Less than 24

[a] Source: Reproduced with permission from Conteh L et al. (4).
The published sources from which these tables are based should be consulted for details of the costs involved.

REFERENCES

1. *The global burden of disease: 2004 update*. Geneva, World Health Organization, 2008.
2. Ramaiah KD et al. The economic burden of lymphatic filariasis in India. *Parasitology Today*, 2000, 16:151-253.
3. Momson JH, Kinnard V, eds. *Different places, different voices*. London, Routledge, 1993.
4. Conteh L, Engels T, Molyneux D. Socioeconomic aspects of neglected tropical diseases. *Lancet*, 2010, 375:239–247.
5. Montresor A et al. Estimation of the cost of large-scale school deworming programmes with benzimidazoles. *Transactions of the Royal Society of Tropical Medicine and Hygiene*, 2010, 104:129–132.

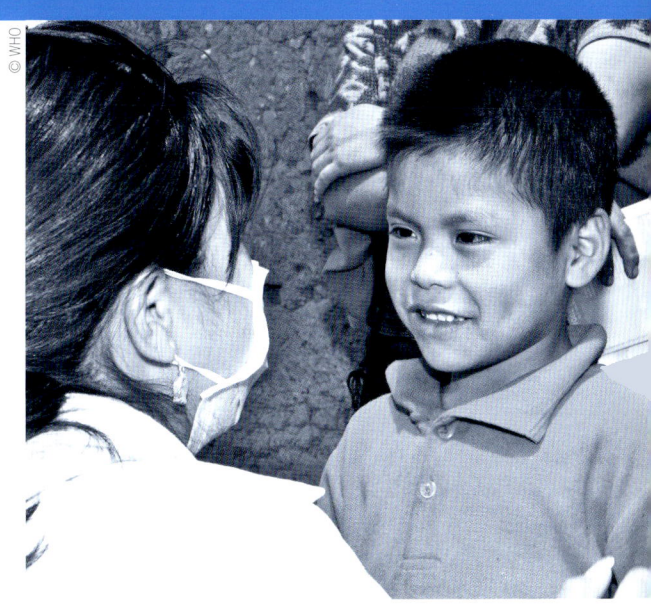

4 Ways forward

4.1 Approaches to overcoming neglected tropical diseases

WHO recommends five strategies for the prevention and control of NTDs: (i) preventive chemotherapy; (ii) intensified case-management; (iii) vector control; (iv) provision of safe water, sanitation and hygiene; and (v) veterinary public health. Working to overcome individual NTDs or a group of these diseases should rely on a combination of the five strategic approaches. For example, in order to control the morbidity caused by lymphatic filariasis, individuals will benefit from preventive chemotherapy; individuals with hydrocoele will require case-management. Bringing the vectors of *Wuchereria* and *Brugia* under control will require appropriate management of water resources. The SAFE strategy (Surgery, Antibiotic treatment, Facial cleanliness and Environmental improvement) used to control trachoma combines the large-scale distribution of medicines with individual case-management and environmental improvement. Surgery for trichiasis prevents progression to blindness. Azithromycin or tetracycline eye ointment offered to populations at risk cures the infection and reduces person-to-person transmission.

WHO fosters technical expertise in each strategy. Sustaining the health benefits will require integration and implementation of the strategies within the national health programmes of countries where NTDs are endemic. This vision is encapsulated in most if not all of the resolutions of the World Health Assembly pertaining to NTDs (*Annex 1*) irrespective of specific, measurable public-health targets.

4.1.1 Preventive chemotherapy

Developed by WHO to control morbidity in populations at risk of infection or illness, preventive chemotherapy depends on the large-scale distribution of high-quality, safety-tested medicines. Preventive chemotherapy is the main intervention for controlling lymphatic filariasis, onchocerciasis, schistosomiasis and soil-transmitted helminthiases. This intervention contributes to the control of trachoma and, depending on the choice of medicine, relieves strongyloidiasis, scabies and lice.

The application of preventive chemotherapy as a public-health measure to control helminthiasis depends on the mass distribution of seven broad-spectrum anthelminthic medicines: albendazole, diethylcarbamazine, ivermectin, levamisole, mebendazole, praziquantel and pyrantel (*Table 4.1.1.1*). WHO recommends these medicines be used not only because of their ease of administration and efficacy but also because of their excellent safety profiles and minimal side-effects (*1*). The safety record of these medicines when used for preventive chemotherapy is such that individual diagnosis is not justified in areas of high endemicity. These medicines are administered as a single, oral dose, either as a single-dose tablet (e.g. albendazole 500 mg or mebendazole 400 mg) or as a dose calculated according to weight or height (dose poles are used to calculate doses for ivermectin and praziquantel). As a result, non-medically trained people, including schoolteachers and community volunteers, can be recruited to deliver these medicines to many people who are beyond the reach of the peripheral health-care system (*2*). The frequency of administration ranges from once to twice yearly, according to the prevailing epidemiology of the targeted infections. Preventive chemotherapy using azithromycin to control morbidity in trachoma forms an effective component of the SAFE strategy. Guidance on the optimum use of preventive chemotherapy under a range of conditions is explained in WHO's manual on preventive chemotherapy in human helminthiasis (*3*).

Table 4.1.1.1 WHO-recommended anthelminthic medicines for use in preventive chemotherapy[a,b,c]

	Disease	Albendazole	Mebendazole	Diethyl-carbamazine	Ivermectin	Praziquantel	Levamisole[d]	Pyrantel[d]
Target diseases for which a well-defined strategy is available	Ascariasis	√	√	–	(√)	–	√	√
	Hookworm	√	√	–	–	–	√	√
	Lymphatic filariasis	√	–	√	√	–	–	–
	Onchocerciasis	–	–	–	√	–	–	–
	Schistosomiasis				–	√	–	–
	Trichuriasis	√	√	–	(√)	–	(√)[e]	(√)[e]
Target diseases for which a strategy is being developed	Clonorchiasis	–	–	–	–	√	–	–
	Opisthorchiasis	–	–	–	–	√	–	–
	Paragonimiasis	–	–	–	–	√	–	–
	Strongyloidiasis	√	(√)	–	√	–	–	–
	Taeniasis	–	–	–	–	√ up to 10 mg/kg	–	–
Additional benefits	Cutaneous larva migrants (zoonotic ancylostomiasis)	√	(√)	–	(√)	–	(√)	(√)
	Ectoparasitic infections (scabies and lice)	–	–	–	√	–	–	–
	Enterobiasis	√	√	–	(√)	–	(√)	√
	Intestinal trematodiases	–	–	–	–	√	–	–
	Visceral larva migrants (toxocariasis)	–	–	√	(√)	–	–	–

[a] Source: adapted from *Preventive chemotherapy in human helminthiasis* (3).

[b] Prescribing information and contraindications are given in the *WHO model formulary 2004*.

[c] In this table, √ indicates medicines recommended by WHO for treatment of the relevant disease, and (√) indicates medicines that are not recommended for treatment but that have a (suboptimal) effect against the disease.

[d] At present, levamisole and pyrantel do not have a prominent role in preventive chemotherapy as described in this manual. However, they remain useful drugs for treating soil-transmitted helminthiases, and since – unlike albendazole and mebendazole – they do not belong to the benzimidazole group, they are expected to contribute to the management of drug-resistant soil-transmitted helminthiases should that problem emerge.

[e] Levamisole and pyrantel have only a limited effect on trichuriasis but, when used in combination with oxantel, pyrantel has an efficacy against trichuriasis comparable to that observed with mebendazole.

Progress towards including preventive chemotherapy in control programmes has been made in some endemic countries, but a considerable scale up will be needed if targets set in resolutions of the World Health Assembly are to be met (*Annex 1*). Global coverage of preventive chemotherapy for the specific forms of helminthiasis is shown in *Figure 4.1.1.1*. The coverage rates are based on information that is available from WHO's preventive chemotherapy and transmission control databank (*4*). A clear difference is noticeable between the rates of coverage for onchocerciasis, lymphatic filariasis, schistosomiasis and soil-transmitted helminthiases. The quality and completeness of data are better for onchocerciasis and lymphatic filariasis, probably because the medicines used to treat these diseases are available in sufficient quantities as part of donations made by the private sector. For reporting purposes, countries are required to submit detailed progress reports before the next year's supply of donated drugs can be granted.

For soil-transmitted helminthiases and schistosomiasis, the situation is different. Even though a large proportion of the population affected by soil-transmitted helminthiases receives albendazole through the Global Programme to Eliminate Lymphatic Filariasis, there is a need to purchase large quantities of generic medicines for reaching persons affected by this disease in areas where lymphatic filariasis is not endemic. Given the large quantities of medicine needed to achieve the required coverage for schistosomiasis and soil-transmitted helminthiases, and the strict timing required for the medicines to be available at the country level, some form of centralized drug supply mechanism should be established, as it is for vaccines supplied for routine immunization.

In fact, preventive chemotherapy for schistosomiasis and soil-transmitted helminthiases may have higher coverage than that shown in *Table 4.1.1.2*. The reported low coverage may be explained by difficulties encountered in collecting and managing data. Since many community-based treatments for schistosomiasis and soil-transmitted helminthiases are delivered by a diverse range of organizations and nongovernmental development organizations, there is a need for greater coordination in reporting. Coverage data are not systematically reported to national authorities by all implementing agencies and are not routinely sent on to the regional and global level of WHO, leading to an underestimation of the numerator. The denominator in calculating coverage may not always be reliable for soil-transmitted helminthiases and particularly for schistosomiasis, which is a highly focal disease.

Fig. 4.1.1.1 Global coverage (%)[a] of preventive chemotherapy for schistosomiasis, soil-transmitted helminthiases, lymphatic filariasis and onchocerciasis[b]

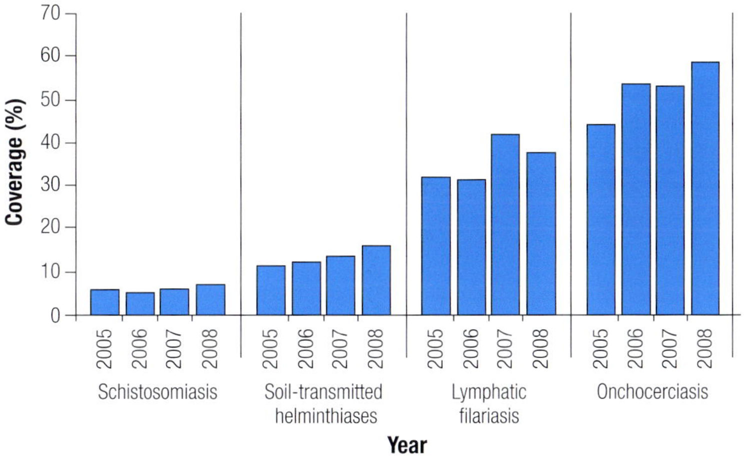

[a] Coverage shown is the proportion of the global population requiring preventive chemotherapy with the appropriate package of medicine for each helminthic infection that has been treated annually between 2005 and 2008. For soil-transmitted helminthiases, the target population is children aged 1–15 years.

[b] Source: *WHO preventive chemotherapy and transmission control databank* (available at: http://www.who.int/neglected_diseases/preventive_chemotherapy/databank/en/).

Table 4.1.1.2 Number of people reached by preventive chemotherapy for at least one neglected tropical disease, 2008

WHO region	Number of countries reporting to WHO	Number of people reached by preventive chemotherapy for at least one disease
African	34	167 575 966
Americas	16	10 987 288
Eastern Mediterranean	7	14 986 795
European	1	37 319
South-East Asia	9	437 651 823
Western Pacific	8	36 831 068
Global	75	668 070 259

4.1.2 Intensified case-management

Intensified case-management involves caring for infected individuals and those at risk of infection. The key processes are (i) making the diagnosis as early as possible, (ii) providing treatment to reduce infection and morbidity, and (iii) managing complications. This intervention is justified as a principal strategy for controlling and preventing those NTDs for which there are no medicines available for preventive chemotherapy. Infection may be asymptomatic for long periods and require confirmation of diagnosis because of the toxicity of medicines. WHO focuses on the prevention and control of Buruli ulcer, Chagas disease, human African trypanosomiasis, leishmaniasis (in its cutaneous, mucocutaneous and visceral forms), leprosy and yaws. For Chagas disease, human African trypanosomiasis and visceral leishmaniasis, diagnosis needs to be simplified and made less invasive without losing sensitivity. For these six and other NTDs, there is an urgent need to shorten the length of time that occurs between suspecting infection and making the diagnosis so that treatment can begin without delay. Innovative work is required to improve diagnostic methods and provide safer medicines for administration under shorter treatment regimens.

The medicines for treatment of the six target diseases include nifurtimox and benznidazole for Chagas disease; pentamidine, suramin, melarsoprol, eflornithine and nifurtimox for human African trypanosomiasis; pentavalent antimonials (sodium stibogluconate and meglumine antimoniate), amphotericin B, paromomycin and miltefosine for visceral leishmaniasis; multidrug therapy for leprosy using a combination of rifampicin, clofazimine and dapsone for multibacillary leprosy, and rifampicin and dapsone for paucibacillary leprosy; a combination of rifampicin and streptomycin or amikacin for Buruli ulcer; and benzathine penicillin for yaws. Most of these medicines are donated to WHO, facilitating the delivery of high-quality treatment free of charge to targeted populations in endemic areas.

4.1.3 Vector control

Vector-borne diseases account for about 16% of the estimated global burden of communicable diseases (5). Most NTDs involve vector transmission: insects transmit the infectious agents of dengue and other virus-induced diseases, Chagas disease, human African trypanosomiasis, leishmaniasis, lymphatic filariasis and onchocerciasis; snails are essential in transmitting the agents of foodborne trematodiasis and schistosomiasis; crustaceans are essential for transmission of the agents of dracunculiasis and foodborne paragonimiasis. Understanding vector biology is an essential component for explaining and predicting the epidemiology of vector-borne disease.

The promotion of integrated vector management is a component of the *Global plan to combat neglected tropical diseases 2008–2015* (6). This approach to vector control requires a rational decision-making process to optimize the use of resources. Effective integrated vector management will be strengthened through close collaboration within sectors responsible for health, agriculture, irrigation and the environment. Several countries where NTDs are endemic have conducted assessments for vector control, and have developed national plans for integrated vector management.

The judicious use of pesticides is important for the control of vector-borne diseases. Deployment of these chemicals has increased significantly, and more than 4000 tonnes of active ingredients (AI) of organochlorine, 800 tonnes (AI) of organophosphate and 230 tonnes (AI) of pyrethroids have been used annually in recent times. Use of such substances on such a scale requires capacity strengthening for the sound management of pesticides from production to disposal of pesticide waste and containers. In the African Region, for example, indoor residual application of pesticide for malaria prevention and control has almost doubled, from reaching 12.5 million to 25 million people during 2005 to 2008.

A survey carried out by WHO in 2003 on the management of public health pesticides by Member States revealed an inadequacy of capacity and legislation for their sound management in some countries (7). The WHO Pesticide Evaluation Scheme (WHOPES) serves as the focal point for pesticide management. WHOPES in collaboration with the Food and Agriculture Organization of the United Nations (FAO) and the United Nations Environment Programme (UNEP) promotes and supports Member States in safe, judicious and effective use of public health pesticides. This includes provision of recommendations on efficacy and safety of public health pesticides and specifications for their quality control and that of application equipment.

Management of pesticides is further complicated by poor coordination between health and agriculture sectors. Substandard pesticides are available, undermining control activities and posing risks to human health and the environment. The variety of pesticides acceptable for use in public health programmes is being depleted, and fewer new products are being launched. The lack of clear career paths for entomologists in health systems in many Member States poses serious difficulties to carrying out effective vector-borne disease control and threatens to impede efforts to sustain progress made in the control of NTDs.

4.1.4 Safe water, sanitation and hygiene

Statistics compiled by the United Nations reveal that 900 million people lack access to safe drinking-water, and 2 500 million lack access to appropriate sanitation (8). Despite the obvious health benefits that accrue from improved sanitation, the targets set under MDG 7 (*Annex 2*) are far from being met, especially in the African and South-East Asia regions. Until this situation improves, many NTDs and other communicable diseases will not be eliminated, and certainly not eradicated. The development and transmission of nine of the NTDs reviewed in this report are related to water and sanitation (9). The situation is emphasized in the flow chart (*Figure 4.1.4.1*).

Fig. 4.1.4.1 Interconnectedness of water and sanitation and the transmission of infectious agents of neglected tropical diseases[a]

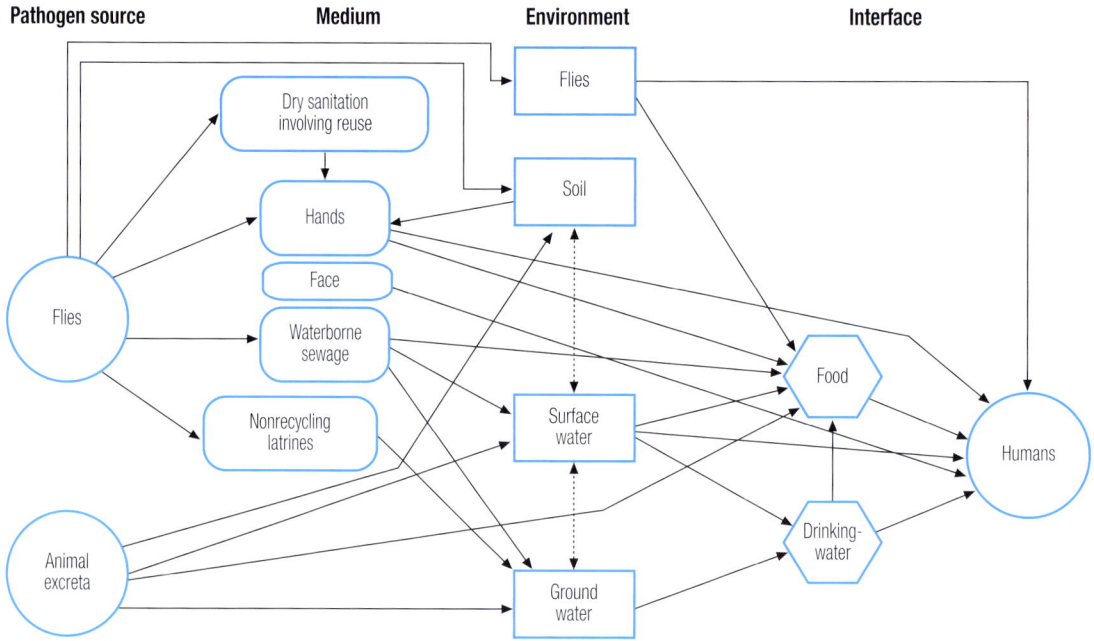

[a] Source: Adapted from Prüss A et al (9).

4.1.5 Veterinary public health: zoonotic aspects of neglected tropical diseases

Veterinary public health is defined as the sum of all contributions to the physical, mental and social well-being of humans through an understanding and application of veterinary sciences (10). The information summarized in section 5 makes clear that much of the morbidity and mortality resulting from NTDs has a major zoonotic component. Zoonotic diseases (zoonoses) are those diseases arising from infections transmitted between vertebrate animals and people. The animals may be domesticated (livestock or companion) or wild. NTDs with a zoonotic component – including brucellosis cysticercosis, echinococcosis, foodborne trematodiasis, human African trypanosomiasis, leishmaniasis and rabies as priority neglected zoonoses – are associated with people living in close proximity to animals. Zoonotic diseases are also factors in the persistence of poverty in places where income and productivity depend on animal health. Control of these diseases in livestock requires interventions that do not threaten the economic security of populations whose livelihoods are dependent on animals. There is a crucial role for veterinarians in the public-health arena.

4.2 Current policies and strategies

Extracts of reports from recent G8 summit meetings are shown in boxes 4.2.1, 4.2.2 and 4.2.3. The G8 countries are committed to action to relieve the burden of suffering from NTDs, thereby making a significant contribution to the attainment of the MDGs.

Box 4.2.1

34th G8 Summit – Tōyako, Japan, July 2008
Report of the G8 Health Experts Group to the G8 leaders[a]

For the 2008 meeting of G8 leaders, the Japanese Presidency established the G8 Health Experts Group to review and recommend methods to overcome the infectious diseases that continue to challenge and impair human health and development. The Group's report focuses on how the commitment of the G8 to the improvement of health will make a significant contribution to the attainment of the Millennium Development Goals.

Importantly, for the diverse community of agencies working with WHO to overcome NTDs, section 25 of the report states:

"An estimated one billion people are affected by a range of neglected tropical diseases (NTD) which cause substantial health, economic and social burdens in poor countries. Efforts to control or eliminate NTDs need to be invigorated. The G8 will work to support the control or elimination of diseases listed by the WHO through such measures as research, diagnostics and treatment, prevention, awareness-raising and enhancing access to safe water and sanitation. In this regard, by expanding health system coverage, alleviating poverty and social exclusion as well as promoting adequate integrated public health approaches, including through the mass administration of drugs, we will be able to reach at least 75% of the people affected by certain major neglected tropical diseases in the most affected countries in Africa, Asia and Latin America, bearing in mind the WHO Plan. With sustained action for 3–5 years, this would enable a very significant reduction of the current burden with the elimination of some of these diseases."

[a] Tōyako Framework for Action on Global Health: report of the G8 Health Experts Group (available at http://www.mofa.go.jp/policy/economy/summit/2008/doc/pdf/0708_09_en.pdf).

Box 4.2.2

35th G8 Summit – L'Aquila, Italy, July 2009
G8 Leaders Declaration: Responsible leadership for a sustainable future[a]

"We warmly support building a global consensus on maternal, newborn and child health as a way to accelerate progress on the Millennium Development Goals for both maternal and child health, through (i) political and community leadership and engagement; (ii) a quality package of evidence-based interventions through effective health systems; (iii) the removal of barriers to access for all women and children, free at the point of use where countries chose to provide it; (iv) skilled health workers; (v) accountability for results. We encourage the work of the WHO, WB, UNICEF and UNFPA are doing to renew international efforts on maternal and child health. We will implement further efforts towards universal access to HIV/AIDS prevention, treatment, care and support by 2010, with particular focus on prevention and integration of services for HIV/TB. We will combine this with actions to: combat TB and Malaria; address the spread of Neglected Tropical Diseases and work towards completing the task of polio eradication; improve monitoring of emerging infectious diseases. In this regard, we stress the importance of addressing gender inequality."

[a] Responsible leadership for a sustainable future (available at http://www.g8italia2009.it/static/G8_Allegato/G8_Declaration_08_07_09_final,0.pdf).

Box 4.2.3

36th G8 Summit – Muskoka, Canada, June 2010
G8 Muskoka Declaration: Recovery and new beginnings[a]

"We reaffirm our commitment to come as close as possible to universal access to prevention, treatment, care and support with respect to HIV/AIDS. We will support country-led efforts to achieve this objective by making the third voluntary replenishment conference of the Global Fund to Fight AIDS, TB and Malaria in October 2010 a success. We encourage other national and private sector donors to provide financial support for the Global Fund. We commit to promote integration of HIV and sexual and reproductive health, rights and services within the broader context of strengthening health systems. G8 donors also remain steadfast in their support for polio eradication and remain committed to a polio-free world. We continue to support the control or elimination of high-burden Neglected Tropical Diseases (NTDs)."

[a] G8 Muskoka Declaration: recovery and new beginnings (available at http://g8.gc.ca/wp-content/uploads/2010/07/declaration_eng.pdf).

4.2.1 The *Global plan to combat neglected tropical diseases 2008–2015*

In 2007, WHO published the *Global plan to combat neglected tropical diseases 2008–2015* (6). Table 4.2.1.1 summarizes its main elements.

Table 4.2.1.1 Key elements of the *Global plan to combat neglected tropical diseases 2008–2015*

Vision	to achieve cost-effective, ethical and sustainable control of neglected tropical diseases
Principles for action	the right of individuals to health
	the use of existing health systems as a setting for interventions
	a response to neglected diseases coordinated by the health system
	integration of health programmes and equity in delivery
	intensified control of neglected diseases as a component of policies that target the poor
	control to be implemented at country and regional levels
Challenges	the procurement and supply of essential medicines for NTDs
	quantification of the burden of NTDs
	provision of treatment and other interventions free of charge
	establishing a system for delivery of medicines to cover populations
	delivery of multi-intervention packages
	development of new diagnostic tools, medicines and pesticides
	production of current and improved medicines and insecticides
	implementation of integrated vector management
	task of advocating for an intersectoral, interprogrammatic approach to NTD control
	building good systems for surveillance and monitoring
	wildlife component of disease control
Goals and targets	eliminate or eradicate those diseases targeted in resolutions of the World Health Assembly and WHO's Regional Committees
	reduce significantly the burden of diseases not yet targeted for elimination or eradication
	ensure that interventions using novel approaches are available, promoted and accessible for diseases that have inadequate control methods
Strategies for action	assessing the burden of NTDs and zoonoses
	taking an integrated approach and adopting multi-intervention packages for disease control
	strengthening health-care systems and building capacity
	ensuring free and timely access to high-quality medicine, and diagnostic and preventive measures
	providing access to innovation
	strengthening integrated vector management and capacity building
	establishing partnerships and mobilizing resources
	developing strategy at country level and regional level

4.2.2 Neglected tropical diseases and the Millennium Development Goals

In 2001, Member States of the United Nations proclaimed and adopted eight Millennium Development Goals (MDGs) (*Annex 2*). The aim of these goals serve to inspire and encourage governments, agencies, institutions and individuals to act so that populations in need will receive support and care.

In response to World Health Assembly resolutions and other initiatives, WHO and its partners in the NTD community are helping to make progress towards achieving the MDG outcomes (*Table 4.2.2.1*). For example, treating school-aged children for schistosomiasis and soil-transmitted helminthiases helps to improve their nutritional status and educational attainment (MDGs 3, 4, 5 and 6). Controlling and eliminating human African trypanosomiasis and onchocerciasis have improved health and contributed to agricultural productivity (MDGs 1 and 4). Such outcomes, if sustained, will make a positive contribution to development, and it is development that will ensure economic growth and that the resources and infrastructure that health care requires are provided.

Table 4.2.2.1 The contribution of the control of neglected tropical diseases (NTDs) to attaining health in the Millennium Development Goals[a] (MDGs) – excerpts from World Health Assembly (WHA) resolutions and other relevant resolutions

	Public health problem	Selected WHA resolutions[b] and other relevant resolutions	Title	Year	MDG associated with NTDs
1	Dracunculiasis	WHA57.9 (Recalling WHA50.35, WHA44.5)	Eradication of dracunculiasis	2004	1, 6
		WHA42.29 (Recalling WHA39.21)	Elimination of dracunculiasis	1989	1, 6
2	Lymphatic filariasis	EM/RC47/R.11	Elimination of lymphatic filariasis in the Eastern Mediterranean Region	2000	6, 8
		WHA50.29	Elimination of lymphatic filariasis as a public health problem	1997	6
		WHA43.18	Tropical disease research	1990	4, 6, 8
		WHA42.31	Control of disease vectors and pests	1989	1, 7, 8
3	Onchocerciasis	WHA47.32	Control of onchocerciasis through ivermectin distribution	1994	6
		WHA42.31	Control of disease vectors and pests	1989	1, 7
4	Schistosomiasis	WHA54.19	Schistosomiasis and soil-transmitted helminth infections	2001	3–8
5	Soil-transmitted helminthiases	WHA54.19	Schistosomiasis and soil-transmitted helminth infections	2001	3–8
6	Taeniasis/Cysticercosis	WHA31.48	Prevention and control of zoonoses and foodborne diseases due to animal products	1978	1, 6, 8
7	Human echinococcosis	WHA31.48	Prevention and control of zoonoses and foodborne diseases due to animal products	1978	1, 6, 8
8	Blinding trachoma	WHA51.11	Global elimination of blinding trachoma	1998	1, 3–8
9	Fascioliasis	WHA31.48	Prevention and control of zoonoses and foodborne diseases due to animal products	1978	1, 6, 8
10	Yaws	WHA31.58	Control of endemic treponematoses	1978	1, 6
11	Dengue	SEA/RC61/R5	Dengue prevention and control	2008	6, 8
		WPR/RC59.R6	Dengue fever and dengue haemorrhagic fever prevention and control	2008	6, 8
		WHA55.17	Prevention and control of dengue fever and dengue haemorrhagic fever	2002	6, 8
		CD43.R4	Dengue and dengue haemorrhagic fever	2001	6, 8
12	Rabies	CD48.R13	15th Inter-American Meeting at ministerial level on health and agriculture (RIMSA): "Agriculture and health: Alliance for equity and rural development in the Americas"	2008	6
		WHA31.48	Prevention and control of zoonoses and foodborne diseases due to animal products	1978	6, 8

Table 4.2.2.1 (continued)

	Public health problem	Selected WHA resolutions[b] and other relevant resolutions	Title	Year	MDG associated with NTDs
13	Cutaneous and mucocutaneous leishmaniasis	WHA60.13	Control of leishmaniasis	2007	3, 6, 7
	Visceral leishmaniasis	WHA60.13	Control of leishmaniasis	2007	3, 4, 6, 8
14	Leprosy	WHA44.9 (Recalling WHA40.35)	Leprosy	1991	1, 6
15	Buruli ulcer	WHA57.1	Surveillance and control of *Mycobacterium ulcerans* disease (Buruli ulcer)	2004	1, 2, 4, 8
16	Chagas disease	WHA63.20	Chagas disease: control and elimination (Recalling resolution CD49.R19 adopted by the 49th Directing Council of PAHO in 2009)	2010	1, 4–6, 8
		WHA51.14	Elimination of transmission of Chagas disease	1998	1, 4–6, 8
17	Human African trypanosomiasis	WHA57.2	Control of human African trypanosomiasis	2004	1, 2, 7, 8
		WHA56.7	Pan African tsetse and trypanosomiasis eradication campaign	2003	1, 2, 7, 8
		WHA50.36	African trypanosomiasis	1997	1, 2, 7, 8

[a] The Millennium Development Goals are: 1 – eradicate extreme poverty and hunger; 2 – achieve universal primary education; 3 – promote gender equality and empower women; 4 – reduce child mortality; 5 – improve maternal health; 6 – combat HIV/AIDS, malaria and other diseases; 7 – ensure environmental sustainability; 8 – develop a global partnership for development.

[b] For a complete list of the WHA resolutions on neglected tropical diseases, see *Annex 1*.

In 2005, the United Nations Millennium Project (*11*) published a set of Quick Win interventions that were devised to deliver significant gains towards attaining the MDGs. One relates directly to the prevention and control of schistosomiasis and soil-transmitted helminthiases. This specific quick win aims to "Provide regular annual deworming to all school children in affected areas to improve health and educational outcomes". Resolution WHA54.19 targets all school-aged children regardless of whether they attend school.

4.2.3 Neglected tropical diseases and health-system strengthening

A health system consists of all the organizations, people and actions whose primary intent is to promote, restore or maintain health. The system includes direct health-improving activities and efforts to influence determinants of health.

A health system consists of more than the pyramid of publicly-owned facilities that deliver personal health services. For example, mothers caring for sick children, private health providers, vector-control campaigns, health insurance organizations, and occupational health and safety legislation form part of a health system. Intersectoral action by health staff – for example to encourage a Ministry of Education to promote female education – is a well known determinant of better health.

Growing recognition by the global community of the unacceptable scale and severity of morbidity resulting from NTDs, coupled with changes in thinking about how to prevent and control them, has provided an opportunity to strengthen health systems in the countries where these diseases have such detrimental effects on health and productivity. Summaries of the progress made in the development and practical application of this thinking, and the options it offers for using NTD control to strengthen health systems, are contained in two reports published by WHO (*12, 13*).

WHO advocates the prevention and control of NTDs using the six components (or core building blocks) that will strengthen the health systems of disease-endemic countries (*14*). The components are:

1. delivery of effective, safe, quality-assured health interventions to the individuals and communities who need them, when and where they need them, with the minimum waste of resources;

2. health workforce able to perform responsively, fairly and efficiently to achieve the best health outcomes possible, given the available resources and circumstances (e.g. there should be enough trained and competent staff evenly distributed to meet needs);

3. health information system to ensure the production, analysis, dissemination and use of reliable and timely information on health determinants, health-system performance and health status;

4. ensure equitable access to essential medicines, vaccines and technologies of assured quality, safety, efficacy and cost-effectiveness, and ensure their scientifically sound and cost-effective delivery;

5. establish a health financing system to raise adequate funds for health in ways that ensure people have access to services and are protected from financial catastrophe or impoverishment associated with having to pay for them;

6. leadership and governance to ensure that strategic policy frameworks exist and are combined with effective oversight, coalition-building, regulation, attention to system-design and transparent accountability.

Close collaboration among WHO, countries and partners is beginning to show that the integration of NTD control does strengthen health systems. In 2007, with considerable financial support from the United States Congress, administered by the United States Agency for International Development, a programme began to expand control in communities of selected NTDs in five countries in sub-Saharan Africa (Burkina Faso, Ghana, Mali, Niger and Uganda). This programme began around the same time as awareness was raised that NTD control could be an agent for strengthening health systems. In 2007, towards the end of the first year of the programme, an independent evaluation reported that, while the degree of integration of control of NTDs into the health systems of the five countries was variable (from partial to fully integrated), there was evidence of strengthening through capacity building in the health workforce and through the introduction of monitoring procedures. For example, the distribution of albendazole, ivermectin, praziquantel and azithromycin, totalling about 37 million doses, to people in need would not have been possible without the training of more than 100 000 people.

The now widely used arrangements for treating children for schistosomiasis and soil-transmitted helminthiases through delivery at primary schools also gives opportunities for health education. Providing instruction to people on how to care for relatives or others in their community suffering from disabling morbidity from dracunculiasis and lymphatic filariasis strengthens health systems, thereby achieving delivery and equitable access.

The drive to achieve strengthened health-care systems is gaining welcome momentum. Since sustainable NTD control is an element of development, donors and agencies beyond disease-endemic countries – the agents of aid to developing countries – will need to accept that countries must have ownership of their health systems and total control over decisions about the health of their people. This point is well made in the *Paris Declaration on aid effectiveness* (*15*), which includes the following principle: "Developing countries will exercise effective leadership over their development policies ...".

REFERENCES

1. De Silva NR et al. Soil-transmitted helminth infections: updating the global picture. *Trends in Parasitology*, 2003, 19:547–551.
2. Mondadori E et al. Appreciation of school deworming program by parents in Ha Giang Province (Vietnam). *Southeast Asian Journal of Tropical Medicine and Public Health*, 2006, 37(6):1095–1098.
3. *Preventive chemotherapy in human helminthiasis. Coordinated use of anthelminthic drugs in control interventions: a manual for health professionals and programme managers.* Geneva, World Health Organization, 2006.
4. *WHO preventive chemotherapy and transmission control databank*. Geneva, World Health Organization, 2010 (http://www.who.int/neglected_diseases/preventive_chemotherapy/databank/en/index.html; accessed July 2010).
5. *The global burden of disease: 2004 uptdate*. Geneva, World Health Organization, 2008.
6. *Global plan to combat neglected tropical diseases 2008–2015*. Geneva, World Health Organization, 2007 (WHO/CDS/NTD/2007.3).
7. *Public health pesticide management practices by WHO Member States. Report of a survey, 2003–2004*. Geneva, World Health Organization, 2004 (WHO/CDS/WHOPES/GCDPP/2004.7; also available at http://whqlibdoc.who.int/hq/2004/WHO_CDS_WHOPES_GCDPP_2004.7.pdf; accessed March 2010).
8. Stikker A et al. "Water, water everywhere…" Innovations to improve global availability of clean water and sanitation. *Innovations*, 2009, 4(3):29–41.
9. Prüss A et al. Estimating the burden of disease from water, sanitation, and hygiene at a global level. *Environmental Health Perspectives*, 2002, 110:538.
10. *Future trends in veterinary public health: report of a WHO study group*. Geneva, World Health Organization, 2002 (WHO Technical Report Series, No. 907; also available at http://whqlibdoc.who.int/trs/WHO_TRS_907.pdf).
11. *Investing in development: a practical plan to achieve the Millennium Development Goals*. New York, NY, United Nations Millennium Project, 2005.
12. *Intensified control of neglected diseases: report of an international workshop, Berlin, 10–12 December 2003*. Geneva, World Health Organization, 2004 (WHO/CDS/CPE/CEE/2004.45).
13. *Strategic and technical meeting on intensified control of neglected tropical diseases: report of an international workshop, Berlin, 18–20 April 2005*. Geneva, World Health Organization, 2006 (WHO/CDS/NTD/2006.1).
14. *Everybody's business – strengthening health systems to improve health outcomes: WHO's framework for action*. Geneva, World Health Organization, 2007.
15. *Paris Declaration on aid effectiveness*. Paris, Organisation for Economic Co-operation and Development, 2005.

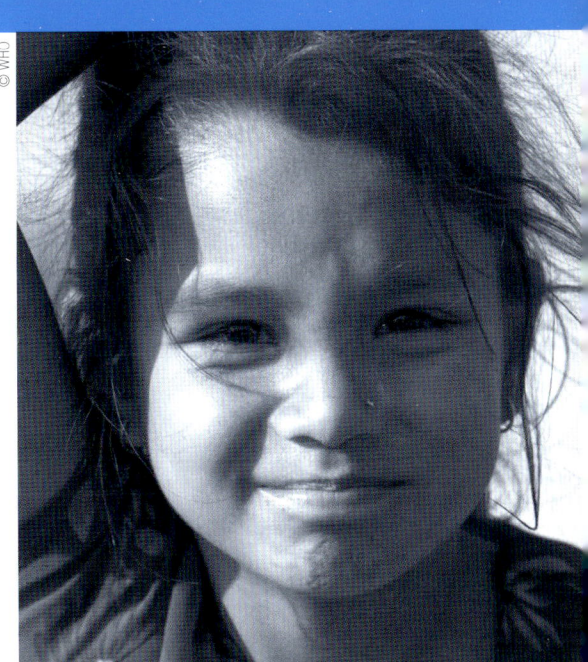

5 Neglected tropical diseases in the world today

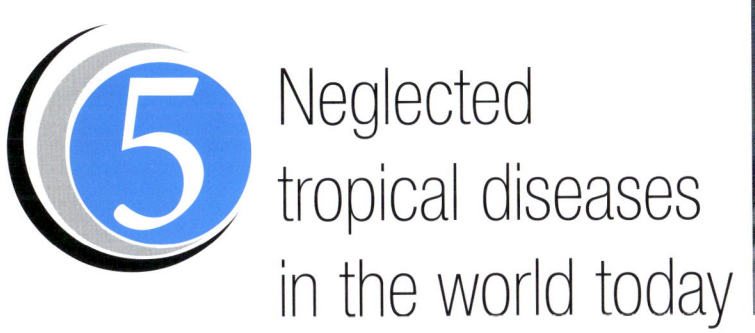

The order in which the information in this section is arranged reflects the increasing molecular and structural complexity of the infectious agents responsible for NTDs. Of the 17 diseases presented in this report, 9 are caused by microparasites (see sections 5.1–5.9) and 8 by macroparasites (see sections 5.10–5.17). This arbitrary classification enabled Anderson and May in 1991 to elucidate principles governing the population dynamics, epidemiology and courses of infection of pathogens that severely impair human health (*1*).

Most microparasites have simple life-cycles and a tendency to replicate within the host. Transmission may be (i) direct, through environmental contamination; (ii) direct, through intimate contact, including the transplacental route; (iii) indirect, through a vector that may or may not be an intermediate host; or (iv) through blood transfusions or organ transplants. The infections microparasites cause range from acute (death or recovery), recurrent (repeated growth and decay of organisms in the host) or inapparent (dormant and difficult to detect) to subclinical (symptomless but detectable).

Macroparasites usually have complex life-cycles involving intermediate and reservoir hosts, and a tendency not to replicate in the definitive human host. Some species of soil-transmitted helminths are an exception in that they do not require intermediate hosts. Transmission may be (i) direct, through ingestion from a contaminated environment; (ii) direct, through skin penetration; (iii) indirect, through ingestion of an infected intermediate host or tissues of a reservoir host; or (iv) indirect, through a vector serving as an intermediate host. The infections caused by macroparasites tend to be chronic rather than acute, and mortality rates are considered low, given the millions of people experiencing disease.

Overcoming infections caused by a number of microparasites and macroparasites is made more difficult because their survival and transmission often exploits a zoonotic component. Zoonotic infections are those in which humans – through behaviour, culture or food supply – have become incorporated into the transmission cycle of pathogens responsible for diseases in wild or domesticated animals.

REFERENCE

1. Anderson RM, May RM. *Infectious diseases of humans: dynamics and control.* Oxford, Oxford University Press, 1991.

5.1 Dengue

Abstract

Dengue results from infection with a virus transmitted mainly by *Aedes aegypti*, a species of mosquito with a global distribution. About 1 million confirmed cases of dengue are reported annually to WHO. Most deaths occur in the South-East Asia Region, where there is a declining trend in the number of reported deaths, and in the Western Pacific Region. There is considerable uncertainty about the actual number of cases given the spread and characteristics of the disease.

Description

Dengue is found in tropical and subtropical regions, predominantly in urban and semi-urban areas. The increase in urban populations is bringing greater numbers of people into contact with *A. aegypti*, especially in areas favourable for mosquito breeding, for example in areas where storing household water is common and where waste disposal services are inadequate.

Dengue haemorrhagic fever – a potentially deadly complication – is characterized by high fever, haemorrhage phenomena (often with enlargement of the liver) and, in severe cases, circulatory failure. The disease, which affects most Asian countries, is a leading cause of hospitalization and death among children in several countries and is widespread in parts of Latin America and the Caribbean.

Distribution and trends

Trends and case-fatality rates discussed in section 5.1 are based on reported cases and therefore may reflect changes in reporting as well as in disease incidence or fatality. Dengue is endemic in all WHO regions except the European Region. Three regions (the Region of the Americas, the South-East Asia Region and the Western Pacific Region) routinely collect information on prevalence and outbreaks of dengue in Member States (*Figure 5.1.1*). The African and Eastern Mediterranean regions also record outbreaks, but the level of endemicity is increasing. The numbers of confirmed cases and deaths are key indicators used by countries to assess the impact of the disease, although national capacities for recording, reporting and classifying cases vary widely.

South-East Asia Region

In 2007, the number of dengue cases reported to WHO from the South-East Asia Region increased by 18% compared with 2006, but it declined in 2008 (*Figure 5.1.2*). The number of severe dengue cases also increased from 2006 to a total of about 250 000 in 2007, including 1966 deaths, although the average case-fatality rate (CFR) for the region is estimated to be less than 1%. In some countries, areas remain where higher CFRs are recorded than the regional and national averages; Indonesia, for example, has geographical areas where the CFR reaches 5% compared with the national average of 1%.

Western Pacific Region

After a major outbreak of dengue in the Western Pacific Region in 1998, the number of reported cases remained at more than 150 000 during 2006–2007 (*Figure 5.1.3*). Between 2000 and 2007, the 8 most affected Pacific island countries and areas were French Polynesia (37 667 cases), Fiji (25 859), New Caledonia (14 270), the Cook Islands (7590), Palau (3146), Wallis and Futuna (2648), American Samoa (2310) and Kiribati (2143). From 1991 to 2004, 72 deaths were reported, most of which occurred during outbreaks in 1998, 2001 and 2003 in Fiji, French Polynesia, New Caledonia, Palau, the Solomon Islands and Tonga. All four serotypes (DEN-1, DEN-2, DEN-3 and DEN-4) have been reported in the Pacific: *A. aegypti* is the main vector, and *A. albopictus* and *A. polynesiensis* are secondary vectors.

Fig. 5.1.1 Number of cases of dengue reported to WHO, 1995–2008

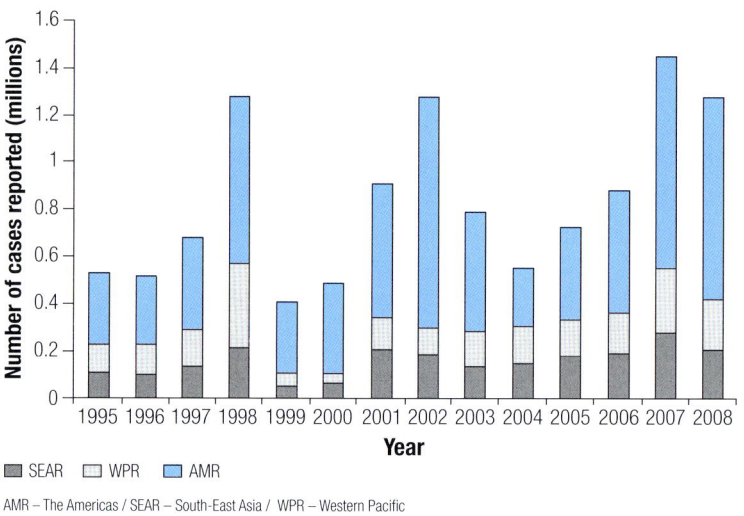

AMR – The Americas / SEAR – South-East Asia / WPR – Western Pacific

Fig. 5.1.2 Number of reported dengue cases and deaths in 11 countries in WHO's South-East Asia Region, 2000–2008 (based on data received by WHO)

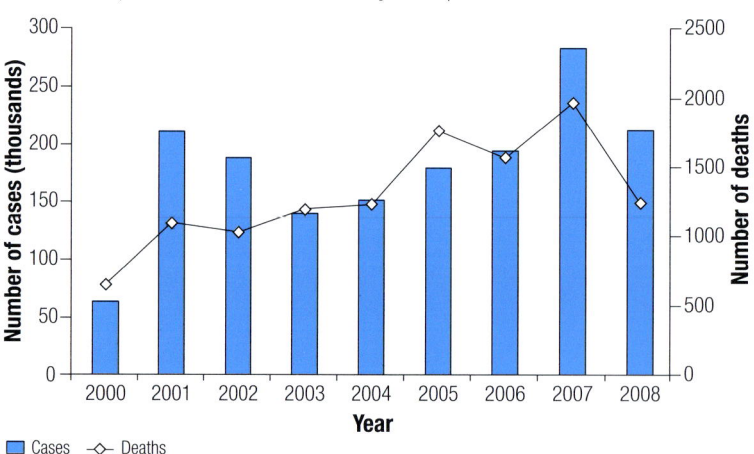

Fig. 5.1.3 Number of reported dengue cases and deaths in 36 countries of WHO's Western Pacific Region, 2000–2008 (based on data received by WHO)

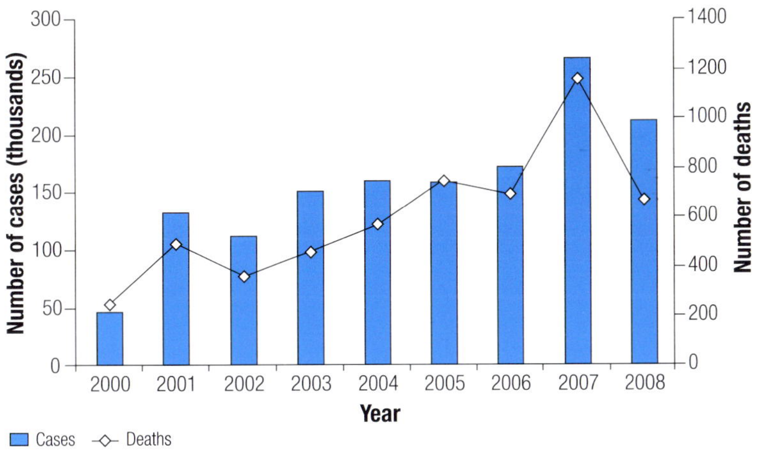

Region of the Americas

The Pan American Health Organization has reported that interruption of dengue transmission in the Region of the Americas resulted from the *A. aegypti* eradication campaign in the region, conducted mainly during the 1960s and early 1970s. Vector surveillance and control measures were not sustained, and subsequent resurgences of *A. aegypti* occurred, followed by dengue outbreaks in the Caribbean and in Central and South America. Dengue has since spread, with outbreaks occurring every 3–5 years. The biggest outbreak – in 2002 – generated more than 1 million reported cases. From 2001 to 2009, more than 30 countries in the Region of the Americas notified a total of 6 626 950 cases of dengue. During the same period, there were 180 216 cases of dengue haemorrhagic fever and 2498 deaths, giving a CFR for dengue haemorrhagic fever of 1.38%. All four serotypes of the virus circulate in the region and were identified simultaneously in 2002 in 10 countries (Barbados, the Bolivarian Republic of Venezuela, Colombia, the Dominican Republic, El Salvador, Guatemala, French Guyana, Mexico, Peru and Puerto Rico). Six countries (the Bolivarian Republic of Venezuela, Brazil, Costa Rica, Colombia, Honduras and Mexico) accounted for over more than 75% of all cases in the region.

Eastern Mediterranean Region

In the Eastern Mediterranean Region, outbreaks of suspected dengue occurred in Pakistan, Saudi Arabia, Sudan and Yemen during 2005–2006 (*1*). In Pakistan, a DEN-3 epidemic of dengue haemorrhagic fever was first reported in 2005 (*2*). Since then, outbreaks have increased in frequency and severity, reaching as far north as the North-West Frontier Province in 2008. Yemen is affected by the increasing frequency and spread of epidemic dengue, and the number of cases has risen since the DEN-3 epidemic in the Western al-Hudeidah governorate in 2005. In 2008, dengue affected the southern province of Shabwa. Since the first death from dengue haemorrhagic fever in Saudi Arabia, in Jeddah in 1993, the country has reported three epidemics: a DEN-2 epidemic in 1994 resulting in 469 cases of dengue, 23 cases of dengue haemorrhagic fever, 2 cases of dengue shock syndrome and 2 deaths; a DEN-1 epidemic in 2006 resulting in 1269 cases of dengue, 27 cases of dengue haemorrhagic fever, 12 cases of dengue shock syndrome and 6 deaths; and a DEN-3 epidemic in 2008 resulting in 775 cases of dengue, 9 cases of dengue haemorrhagic fever, 4 cases of dengue shock syndrome and 4 deaths.

African Region

In the African Region, data from dengue surveillance remain sparse, and cases and outbreaks are not reported to WHO regularly. During 1984–1985, the first major outbreak of DEN-3 was documented in Pemba, Mozambique. Most patients experienced secondary infections and 2 deaths were attributed to dengue haemorrhagic fever. DEN-3 was identified again in a mixed outbreak caused by DEN-2 and DEN-3 in Somalia in 1993 (*3*). Subsequent dengue outbreaks have been reported from different countries, for example Senegal (1999, DEN-2); DEN-3 cases were confirmed in Côte d'Ivoire in 2006 and 2008 (*3*). In October 2009, a major outbreak of DEN-3 in Cape Verde caused 5985 cases and 6 deaths (*4*).

Fig. 5.1.4 Distribution of countries or areas at risk of dengue transmission, worldwide, 2008

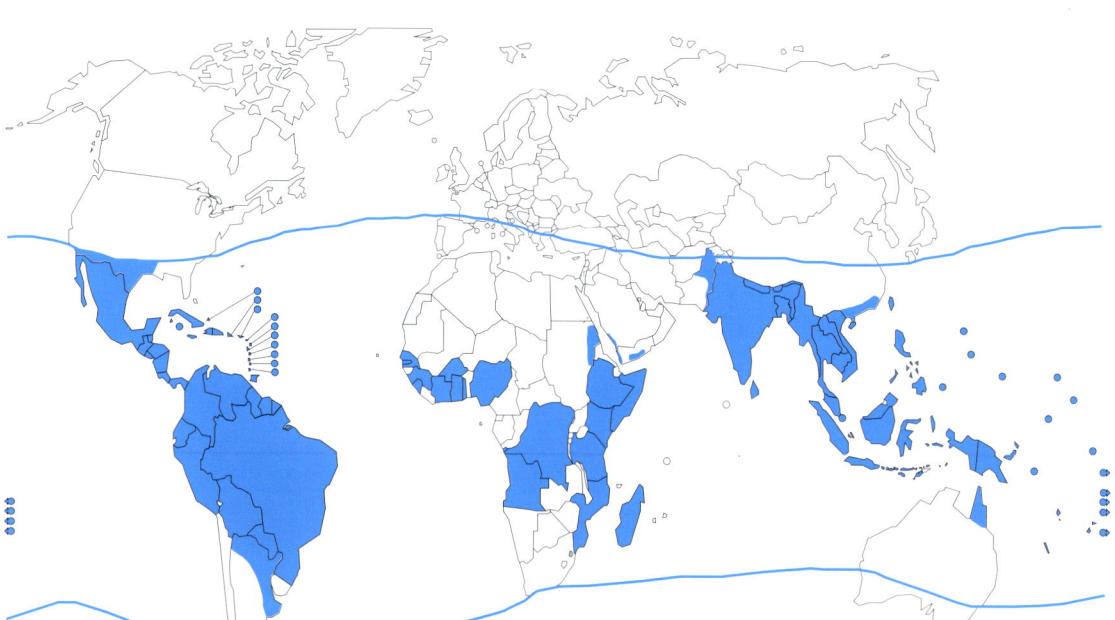

Transmission

The serotypes of the dengue virus are transmitted through the bites of infected *Aedes* mosquitoes, principally *A. aegypti*. This mosquito is widely distributed, mostly between latitudes 35 °N and 35 °S. These geographical limits correspond approximately to a winter isotherm of 10 °C (*Figure 5.1.4*). Its occurrence is relatively uncommon at higher than 1000 metres due to lower temperatures. The immature larval stages are found in water-filled habitats, mostly in artificial containers closely associated with human dwellings, and often indoors. Dengue outbreaks have also been attributed to *A. albopictus*, *A. polynesiensis* and several species of the *A. scutellaris* complex. Each species has a particular ecology, behaviour and geographical distribution. Since the 1980s, *A. albopictus* has spread from Asia to Africa, the Americas and Europe, notably aided by the international trade in used tyres into which mosquito eggs were deposited when they contained rainwater.

A cycle of sylvatic transmission has been identified in West Africa, where DEN-2 has been found circulating among monkeys (*Erythrocebus patas*) and sylvatic *Aedes* species, including *A. taylori*, *A. furcifer* and *A. luteocephalus*.

Since 2007, more than 1 million confirmed cases of dengue have been reported annually to WHO from three regions (the Region of the Americas and the South-East Asia and Western Pacific regions); more than 60% of cases are reported from the Region of the Americas. Some estimates indicate that 50 million cases may now occur every year, of which 8 million are clinical cases (5), and that dengue is spreading globally. The South-East Asia Region accounts for most deaths, but CFRs have shown a downward trend since 2007. This decline has been attributed mainly to effective training in standardized case-management that is based on a network of expertise and training materials.

Economic impact

The aggregated annual economic cost of dengue – based on multicentre studies in 8 countries (the Bolivarian Republic of Venezuela, Brazil, Cambodia, El Salvador, Guatemala, Malaysia, Panama and Thailand) – was estimated to be at least US$ 587 million. Preliminary adjustment for underreporting could raise this total to US$ 1 800 million (6).

Prevention and control

Environmental management and vector control using insecticides are the main approaches for dengue prevention. In 2007, 26 countries from the Americas, South-East Asia and Western Pacific regions reported to WHO on the use of insecticides for dengue vector control. More than 222 tonnes of active ingredient of organophosphate and 27 tonnes of active ingredients of pyrethroid insecticides were used. Such applications are used for larviciding, space spraying and perifocal residual spraying.

In 1995, WHO developed a strategy for dengue prevention and control based on (i) selective integrated vector control, with community and intersectoral participation; (ii) active disease surveillance based on a strong health information system; (iii) emergency preparedness; (iv) capacity building and training; and (v) research into vector control. Successful programmes based on integrated vector management and intersectoral collaboration are being implemented in Cuba, Malaysia and Singapore. Sustaining such integrated vector management activities and implementing them in other settings are the main challenges. The integrated management strategy for dengue prevention and control has been approved by 19 countries in the Region of the Americas. In 2009, WHO published revised guidelines on dengue prevention and control, including case-management (*7*), which recommend follow-up training activities at regional and national levels.

Assessment

Outbreaks of dengue are increasing and spreading geographically. In 2008, Member States of the South-East Asian and Western Pacific Regions adopted resolutions on dengue fever. In response to dengue epidemics, WHO recommends selective vector control, active disease and vector surveillance and management of severe cases in accordance with WHO's guidelines (*7*). Sustained prevention of dengue requires widespread vector control, environmental management and possibly the development of a vaccine.

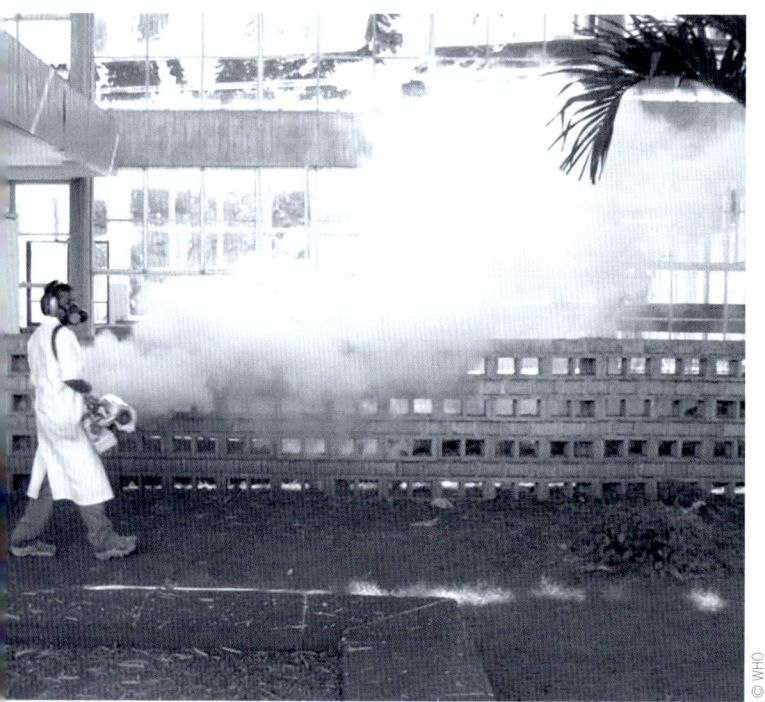

Space-spraying activity outside a public building during a chikungunya outbreak in Mauritius, 2006. Timely and proper space-spray application of insecticides is useful in reducing transmission of dengue and chikungunya.

REFERENCES

1. Spread of dengue fever: the challenges. *DCD Newsletter*, 2005, 6:7–8 (also available at http.//www.emro.who.int/pdf/dcdnewsletter6.pdf).
2. Bushra J et al. Dengue virus serotype 3, Karachi, Pakistan. *Emerging Infectious Diseases*, 2007, 13(1):182–183.
3. Dengue in Africa: emergence of DENV-3, Côte d'Ivoire, 2008. *Weekly Epidemiological Record*, 2009, 84:85–96.
4. Dengue fever, Cape Verde. *Weekly Epidemiological Record*, 2009, 84:469.
5. *The global burden of disease: 2004 update.* Geneva, World Health Organization, 2008.
6. Suayaja et al. Cost of dengue cases in eight countries in the Americas and Asia: a prospective study. *American Journal of Tropical Medicine and Hygiene*, 2009, 80:846–855.
7. *Dengue: guidelines for diagnosis, treatment, prevention and control.* Geneva, World Health Organization, 2009 (WHO/HTM/NTD/DEN/2009.1).

5.2 Rabies

Abstract

Rabies is caused by a virus that is maintained in nature by many wild and domestic carnivore host species as well as bats. The disease is transmitted mainly through bites. Once symptoms develop, the disease is almost 100% fatal. In humans, clinical disease can be prevented through timely immunization even after exposure to the infective agent. Rabies infection causes tens of thousands of deaths every year. Most of these deaths occur in Africa and Asia following dog bites. Every year, more than 15 million people receive post-exposure prophylaxis after being bitten by a suspected rabid animal. Most deaths from human rabies in developing countries can be prevented through interventions directed at dogs, which are the main host and reservoir of the disease.

Description

Rabies is transmitted to other susceptible animals and humans through infectious saliva from rabid animals via transdermal bites, scratches, or licks to broken skin or mucous membranes. In rare instances, the disease may be contracted by inhalation of virus-containing aerosol or via infected organ transplants.

The incubation period usually lasts 1–3 months but may vary from less than 1 week to more than 1 year. Initial symptoms are usually nonspecific and suggest involvement of the respiratory, gastrointestinal and/or central nervous systems. In the acute stage, signs of hyperactivity (furious rabies) or paralysis (dumb rabies) predominate. In both furious and dumb rabies, paralysis eventually progresses to complete paralysis followed by coma and death in all cases, usually as a result of respiratory failure. Without intensive care, death occurs during the first 7 days of illness.

Rabies is widely distributed across the globe, with only a few countries (mainly islands and peninsulas) being free of the disease (*Figure 5.2.1*). Many animal species are involved in the maintenance and transmission of the disease in nature. Fox rabies has been brought under control in Western Europe, but skunk, raccoon and fox rabies remain prevalent in parts of Canada and the United States (*1*); jackals, bat-eared foxes and mongoose are involved in rabies transmission in Africa, particularly in the south-eastern part of the continent (*2*). A variety of bat species have been shown to harbour rabies or rabies-related viruses in Africa, Australia, central and south-east Asia, Europe and most of the Americas. Infected wildlife species, including bats, can transmit rabies to humans, but the total number of such cases remains limited compared with the annual number of human deaths caused by dog-transmitted rabies. By contrast, canine rabies predominates in most of the developing countries of central and south America, Africa and Asia, where the greater burden of human rabies falls. More than 90% of cases of human rabies are transmitted by dogs (3); most deaths occur in Asia and Africa (4).

Fig. 5.2.1 Distribution of risk levels for humans contracting rabies, worldwide, 2009

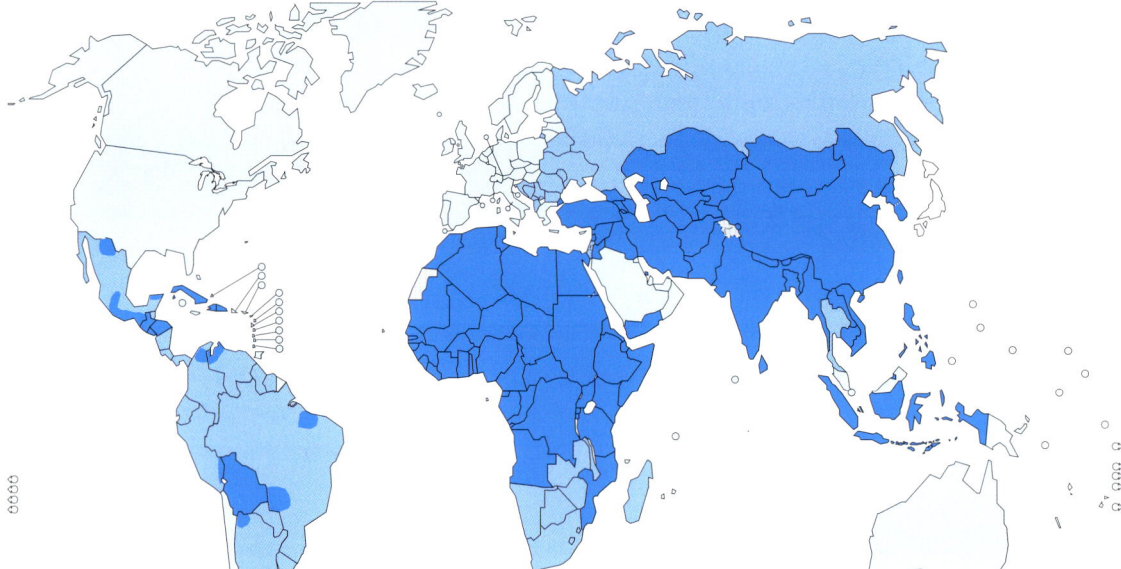

Most African countries report the presence of human and dog rabies in all or large parts of their territories. Information about the public-health impact of wildlife rabies is limited. With some exceptions, data collected at the national level are largely incomplete, notably for human rabies, and are often based on clinical observations rather than laboratory diagnosis (5). A number of African countries have a national plan for controlling rabies through dog immunization and population control, including post-exposure prophylaxis to prevent human rabies. However dog vaccination coverage remains below the required threshold of 70% and the availability of human vaccine is limited, especially in rural areas. Targets for controlling and eliminating human and dog rabies at the regional level have not been established. Since early 2009, South Africa and the United Republic of Tanzania have been working to eliminate human and dog rabies from pilot areas within 5 years.

In Latin American countries, national programmes for controlling dog rabies, which were initiated in 1983 and mainly based on mass immunization of dogs, have stopped dog-to-dog transmission and eliminated human rabies from most urban areas. Dog rabies is, however, still widespread in Cuba, the Dominican Republic, El Salvador, Guatemala, Haiti and the Plurinational State of Bolivia. Rabies in vampire bats is widespread in Latin America; clusters of human deaths associated with contact with bats are regularly reported in the Amazon forest, particularly in Brazil and Peru. Rabies in non-vampire bat species has emerged as a public-health problem in many Latin American countries since 2000. By 2003, the number of cases of dog-transmitted human rabies had fallen by more than 90% (*6*). Since then, fewer than 50 human rabies deaths have been reported annually in the Region of the Americas, the majority still resulting from contact with dogs. In 2008, the 15th inter-American inter-ministerial meeting on health and agriculture set a target for eliminating dog rabies in Latin America by 2012 (*7*). In Canada and the United States, large programmes are under way to control and eliminate rabies in wild carnivore hosts. Cases of human rabies (mostly transmitted by bats) remain rare in both countries.

In the Eastern Mediterranean Region, rabies virus circulates mostly in dogs, but the Islamic Republic of Iran, Oman and Saudi Arabia have reported the involvement of wolves, jackals and foxes. The Islamic Republic of Iran and Sudan provide high numbers of human post-exposure prophylaxis regimens per million inhabitants to prevent the occurrence of human rabies, whereas in Afghanistan, Pakistan and Yemen these numbers are below those expected in countries where rabies is endemic (*8*).

In western Europe during the past 15 years, fox rabies has been eliminated from all affected countries following more than 30 years of mass oral vaccination campaigns in foxes. In 2008, wildlife rabies in foxes and raccoon dogs was still reported in many countries of eastern Europe, such as Belarus, Poland and Ukraine, as well as in the Russian Federation. In south-eastern Europe, fox rabies is present in Slovenia, and rabies occurs in foxes and dogs in Croatia, Bosnia and Herzegovina, Bulgaria, Romania, Montenegro and Serbia (*9*). Only Albania, the Former Yugoslav Republic of Macedonia and Greece reported the absence of rabies to WHO in 2008. The Russian Federation and Turkey reported significant numbers of cases of dog rabies. In the Russian Federation, the dominant epidemiological pattern in the north and south-western part of the country is wildlife rabies involving foxes and raccoon dogs; this is spreading eastwards into Siberia (*10*). In 2003, the Russian Federation launched a new wildlife rabies vaccination project at its northern border with Finland and is planning a similar project with Poland. In 2005, Turkey launched a nationwide project to eliminate dog rabies with support from the European Union. The rabies situation in Azerbaijan, Tajikistan and Uzbekistan is not well known (*11*). In the European Region, the number of human deaths from rabies is estimated to be fewer than 100 cases annually, most of which involve dogs.

Dog rabies is present in all countries of the South-East Asia Region. Data collected at the national level are often based on clinical signs rather than laboratory diagnosis. In India, 20 000 rabies deaths (that is about 2/100 000 population at risk) are estimated to occur annually (*12*). In Thailand and Sri Lanka, national plans for controlling and eliminating dog rabies are in place. Progress is evident in Thailand where 8 human cases of rabies were reported to WHO in 2008 compared with 74 in 1995. Sri Lanka reported 55 cases in 2008 compared with the more than 100 cases reported annually in previous years. In Indonesia, however, dog rabies has spread eastwards to a number of islands since the late 1990s, including Flores in 1998, Maluku in 2003 and Bali in 2008, which historically had been free of rabies (*13*). Nepal has made significant progress in preventing and controlling rabies and now produces its own human and veterinary rabies vaccines.

Japan, New Zealand and smaller island nations in the Pacific Ocean are rabies-free. Bat rabies has been reported in Australia, and is suspected to circulate among bats in other countries in the region including Cambodia, the Philippines and Thailand. In the Republic of Korea – where the last case of human rabies was reported in 2005 – the virus circulates in raccoon dogs. In China, rabies has re-emerged during the past 15 years: more than 2500 deaths were reported in 2004, mostly from 6 south-central provinces; a peak of 3300 deaths occurred in 2007 (*14*). Activities to control dog rabies and better target the delivery of post-exposure prophylaxis have reduced that number of deaths to less than 2500 in 2008. In Viet Nam, rabies was reported in 25/63 provinces in 2007, with clusters of human cases occurring in both northern and southern provinces. Rabies is still widely distributed in the Philippines, where about 250 deaths are reported annually. A number of islands at the centre of the archipelago are aiming to achieve elimination by 2013. A number of rabies-affected Asian countries are committed to eliminating human and dog rabies by 2020 (*15*).

Mortality

Deaths from rabies in humans are considered to be underreported in several countries (*3*). Asia and Africa account for the vast majority of rabies fatalities. Although all age groups are susceptible, rabies is most common in people younger than 15 years; post-exposure prophylaxis is given on average to 40% of children in Asia and Africa aged 5–14 years, and the majority receiving treatment are male. In the north of the United Republic of Tanzania, the incidence of rabies is 3–5 times higher in children younger than 15 years than in adults (*16*).

The most severe injuries, such as multiple head or neck bites, or both, have the shortest incubation period and tend to occur in the youngest children.

Every year, more than 15 million people receive post-exposure prophylaxis, mostly in China and India. In Thailand, the mass vaccination of dogs and widespread use of post-exposure prophylaxis have significantly reduced the number of human deaths from rabies. Post-exposure prophylaxis is thought to prevent more than 270 000 deaths in Asia and Africa (*3*).

Economic impact

Estimating the economic impact of rabies should take into account the costs of post-exposure prophylaxis, the control of rabies in dogs, losses to the livestock industry and surveillance of the disease. Livestock losses can be significant, as indicated by the results of a study carried out in Ethiopia, where it was estimated that deaths among cattle caused by rabies cost the average household US$ 7.50 per year (*17*), equivalent to 7.5% of annual gross national income per capita. The estimated total expenditure for preventing and controlling rabies in Africa and Asia is about US$ 585 million annually. The greater part of the financial burden falls on Asia, with 96% of total rabies expenditure occurring in the region. The breakdown of expenditure by cost category shows that the costs of post-exposure treatment borne by patients form the bulk of expenditure, accounting for nearly half of the total costs attributed to rabies. This expenditure as well as the frequency of delivering post-exposure prophylaxis is expected to rise as all countries, particularly by those replacing nerve-tissue vaccines by imported rabies vaccines developed in cell cultures or embryonated eggs. In Asia and Africa, the cost of human post-exposure treatment represents the main component of the economic burden of rabies; in Latin American countries such as Brazil and Mexico, the cost of interventions aimed at controlling the disease in animals exceeds that of post-exposure treatment. The annual global expenditure for rabies prevention and control exceeds US$ 1 billion, by WHO's conservative assessment.

Prevention and control

Where rabies is a public-health issue, preventing the disease in humans depends on a combination of interventions including controlling rabies in both wild and domestic animals, particularly dogs; providing pre-exposure immunization to humans at occupational risk of contracting the disease; and on delivering post-exposure prophylaxis to potentially exposed patients (*18*). Theoretical and empirical studies show that immunizing 70% of the dog population is required to stop dog-to-dog transmission (*2, 19–21*). The level of success achieved by vaccination programmes depends on knowledge of the ecology of the dog population and the nature of human–dog interactions in the area.

Clinical infection in humans can be prevented by delivering prompt local wound care and the timely administration of post-exposure treatment in the form of rabies immunoglobulin and serial immunizations. Early post-exposure use of vaccines combined with proper wound treatment and administration of rabies immunoglobulin is considered to be nearly 100% effective in preventing death, even with high-risk exposure.

Reducing the burden of rabies and eliminating the disease in humans involve coordinated efforts to procure and deliver safe and efficacious rabies vaccines where they are most needed for preventive immunization in animals and pre-exposure and post-exposure prophylaxis in humans. Awareness of preventive measures is lacking among the general population, even in the most highly endemic regions, and many people exposed to the risk of rabies do not seek care at local health units where rabies biologicals may be available (*16*). Improving the delivery of post-exposure treatment alone does not offer a long-term solution that will prevent deaths, especially among children (*22*). Countries are encouraged to initiate measures that ensure coordination among all public sectors involved in rabies control. Efforts should be coordinated among public sectors concerned with surveillance and reporting, diagnosis, information campaigns, and vaccination of individuals and groups at risk of exposure (*2*).

Assessment

Rabies remains a major public-health and economic concern for ministries of health and agriculture in developing countries. This burden, which is increasing with the continued demand for and consumption of safe and efficacious post-exposure treatment, could be reduced and even eliminated through coordinated interventions aimed at controlling the disease in dogs. To achieve this goal, pilot studies are in progress to demonstrate by 2013 the cost-effectiveness of immunizing dogs in order to prevent rabies in humans.

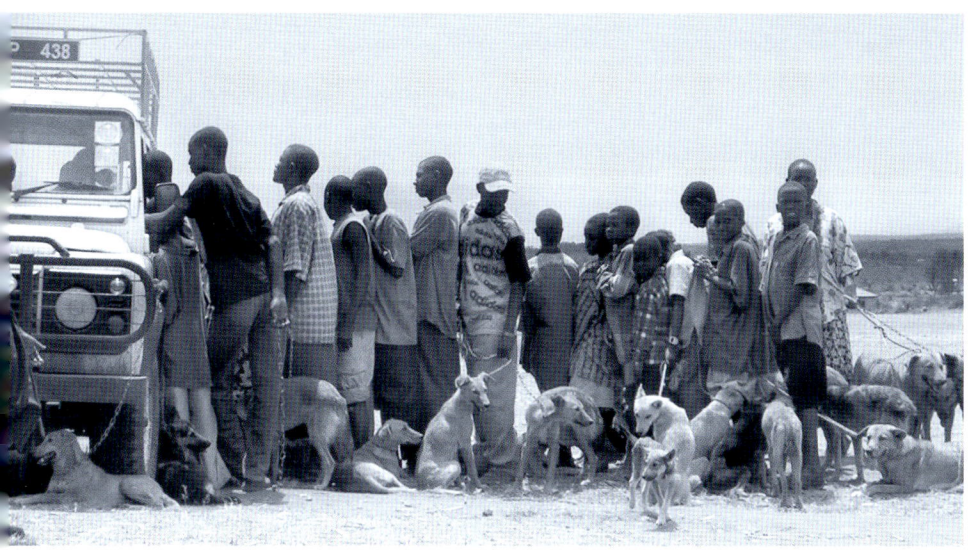

Mass vaccination campaign of dogs, United Republic of Tanzania. Dogs continue to be the main carrier of rabies, particularly in Africa and Asia. Humans most often become infected through the bite or scratch of an infected dog. Mass vaccination of pets helps to prevent occurrence of human rabies.

© Sarah Cleaveland

REFERENCES

1. Rupprecht CE et al. Can rabies be eradicated? *Developments in Biological Standardization (Basel)*, 2008, 131:95–121.
2. Bishop GC. Canine rabies in South Africa. In: Bingham J, Bishop GC, King AA, eds. *Proceedings of the Third International Conference of the Southern and East African Rabies Group, Harare, 7–9 March 1995*. Marcel Merieux Foundation, 1996:104–111.
3. *WHO Expert Consultation on Rabies*. Geneva, World Health Organization, 2005 (WHO Technical Report Series, No. 931).
4. Knobel DL et al. Re-evaluating the burden of rabies in Africa and Asia. *Bulletin of the World Health Organization*, 2005, 83:360–368.
5. Dodet B et al. Fighting rabies in Africa: the Africa Rabies Expert Bureau (AfroREB), *Vaccine*, 2008, 26:6295–6298.
6. Schneider MC et al. Current status of human rabies transmitted by dogs in Latin America. *Cadernos de Saúde*, 2007, 23:2049–2063.
7. *15th inter-American meeting at ministerial level, on health and agriculture*. Rio de Janeiro, Brazil, 11–12 June 2008. World Health Organization/Pan American Health Organization (RIMSA15/1, Rev. 2 (Sp.). 10 December 2007).
8. Seimenis A. The rabies situation in the Middle East. In: Proceedings of a joint OIE/WHO/EU International conference "Towards the elimination of rabies in Eurasia", Paris, France, 27–30 May 2007. *Developments in Biologicals*, 2008, 131:43–53.
9. Wandeler AI. The rabies situation in Western Europe. In: Proceedings of a joint OIE/WHO/EU international conference "Towards the elimination of rabies in Eurasia", Paris, France, 27–30 May 2007. *Developments in Biologicals*, 2008, 131:19–26.
10. Matouch O. The rabies situation in Eastern Europe. In: proceedings of a joint OIE/WHO/EU international conference "Towards the elimination of rabies in Eurasia", Paris, France, 27–30 May 2007. *Developments in Biologicals*, 2008, 131:27–36.
11. Gruzdev KN. The rabies situation in Central Asia. In: Proceedings of a joint OIE/WHO/EU international conference "Towards the elimination of rabies in Eurasia", Paris, France, 27–30 May 2007. *Developments in Biologicals*, 2008, 131:37–42.

12. Sudarshan M et al. Assessing the burden of human rabies in India: results of a national multi-center epidemiological survey. *International Journal of Infectious Diseases*, 2007, 11: 29–35.
13. Windiyaningsih C et al. The rabies epidemic on Flores Island, Indonesia (1998–2003). *Journal of the Medical Association of Thailand*, 2004, 87:1389–1393.
14. Fu ZF. The rabies situation in far East Asia. In: Proceedings of a joint OIE/WHO/EU international conference "Towards the elimination of rabies in Eurasia", Paris, France, 27–30 May 2007. *Developments in Biologicals*, 2008, 131:55–61.
15. *Call for action: towards the elimination of rabies in the ASEAN Member States and the Plus Three Countries*. Jakarta, Association of Southeast Asian Nations.
16. Hampson K et al. Rabies exposures, post-exposure prophylaxis and deaths in a region of endemic canine rabies. *PLoS Neglected Tropical Diseases*, 2008, 2(11):e339.
17. Laurenson MK et al. Rabies as a threat to the Ethiopian wolf (*Canis simensis*). In: Kitala P et al., eds. *Proceedings of 5th meeting of the Southern and Eastern African Rabies Group (SEARG), Nairobi Kenya 4–6 March 1997*. Lyon, Fondation Marcel Merieux, 1998:97–103.
18. Rabies vaccines: WHO position paper. *Weekly Epidemiological Record*, 2010, 85: 309–320.
19. Kitala PM et al. Comparison of vaccination strategies for the control of dog rabies in Machakos District, Kenya. *Epidemiology and Infection*, 2002, 129:215–222.
20. Cleaveland S et al. A dog rabies vaccination campaign in rural Africa: impact on the incidence of dog rabies and human dog-bite injuries. *Vaccine*, 2003, 21:1965–1973.
21. Zinsstag J et al Transmission dynamics and economics of rabies control in dogs and humans in an African city. *PNAS*, 2009, 106:14996–15001.
22. Cleaveland S et al. Canine vaccination-providing broader benefits for disease control. *Veterinary Microbiology*, 2006, 117:53–50.

5.3 Trachoma

Abstract

In 57 countries where trachoma is endemic millions of people have irreversible visual impairment and blindness caused by the disease, and more than 40 million people are in need of treatment. Trachoma is caused by an obligate intracellular microorganism (*Chlamydia trachomatis*), which is transmitted through contact with eye and nose discharge from infected people, particularly children, and, possibly, by eye-seeking flies. The economic cost of trachoma in terms of lost productivity is estimated at US$ 2.9 billion annually. Activities to control the disease should adopt the SAFE strategy – that is, lid surgery (S), antibiotics to treat the community pool of infection (A), facial cleanliness (F) and environmental improvement (E).

Description

Trachoma is responsible for approximately 3% of the world's blindness (*1*). Environmental risk factors influencing transmission of the disease include poor hygiene, crowded households, water shortage and inadequate latrines. After years of repeated infection, the inside of the eyelid may become scarred so severely that it turns inward and the lashes rub the eyeball (trichiasis) and scar the cornea. Left untreated, this condition – called "blinding trachoma" – leads to the formation of irreversible corneal opacities and blindness.

In areas where trachoma is endemic, the average age of acquisition of the first episode of *C. trachomatis* infection is related to the prevailing level of infection in the community: in hyperendemic settings, infection may be acquired in early infancy. Infection is usually acquired through living in close proximity to an infected person, and the family is the principal unit for transmission (*2*).

Distribution

Blinding trachoma is hyperendemic in many of the poorest and most remote rural areas in 57 countries of Africa, Asia, Central and South America, Australia and the Middle-East (*Figure 5.3.1*) (*3*).

Roughly half the global burden of active trachoma is concentrated in 5 countries (Ethiopia, Guinea, India, Nigeria and Sudan), and that of trichiasis in 4 countries (China, Ethiopia, Nigeria and Sudan). Overall, Africa is the most affected continent: 27.8 million cases of active trachoma (68.5% of all cases globally) and 3.8 million cases of trichiasis (46.6% of all) occur in 28/46 countries in the African Region. The highest prevalences of active trachoma have been reported from Ethiopia and Sudan, where the infection often occurs in more than 50% of children younger than 10 years; trichiasis is found in up to 19% of adults.

Fig. 5.3.1 Distribution of trachoma, worldwide, 2009

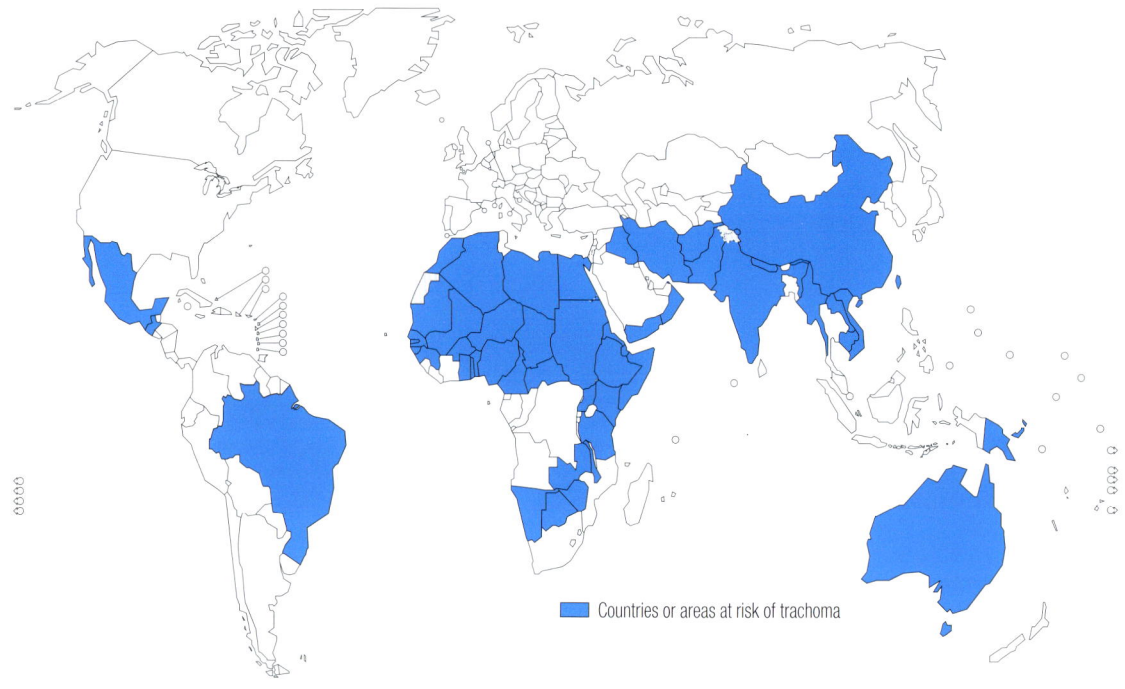

Morbidity

Trichiasis causes additional disability through severe ocular pain every time a person blinks, which adds to the burden of disease (*4*). Studies undertaken in rural communities in sub-Saharan Africa to assess excess mortality caused by visual impairment found an increase in mortality among blind people compared with sighted controls (*5, 6*).

The clinical manifestations of trachoma change with age. In hyperendemic areas, active trachoma is common in preschool-aged children, with prevalence rates as high as 60–90%, but it becomes less frequent and shorter in duration with increasing age (*7*). Epidemiological surveys have generally found trichiasis to be more common in women than in men (*8*). This difference has been attributed to the greater exposure of women to *C. trachomatis* through closer contact with children, the main source of infection. Conjunctival scarring accumulates with age, usually becoming evident in the second or third decade of life (*9*). The onset of blinding complications can occur in children living in regions where the prevalence of infection is high.

Economic impact

The burden of trachoma on affected individuals and communities is considerable in terms of disability and economic costs. Lost productivity has been estimated to cost between US$ 2.9 billion and US$ 5.3 billion per year (*10*), increasing to US$ 8 billion when trichiasis is included.

Prevention and control

Trachoma control programmes in endemic countries are being implemented at a different pace. In 1998, the World Health Assembly resolved to eliminate blinding trachoma as a public-health problem by the year 2020 (*11*). To this end, control activities have been instituted through primary health-care approaches that follow the SAFE strategy, which consists of lid surgery (S), antibiotics to treat the community pool of infection (A), facial cleanliness (F) and environmental improvement (E).

There is evidence to support the effectiveness of each component of the SAFE strategy (*12*). Problems with surgical outcomes may include high rates of trichiasis recurrence reported under operational conditions (*13*). The overall cost-effectiveness of implementing the SAFE strategy has been estimated at US$ 54 per case of visual impairment prevented (*14*, *15*).

Various countries have set target dates for the elimination of blinding trachoma. Member States and partners have agreed to accelerate implementation of the SAFE strategy in order to reflect the planned progression of elimination activities and achieve the relevant elimination targets (*Figure 5.3.2*). It is estimated that, during 2008–2012, about 1.7 billion doses of azithromycin and 19 million tubes of tetracycline eye ointment will be required to treat 60% of the target populations with preventive chemotherapy where trachoma is endemic; the cost is equivalent to approximately US$ 0.4 billion.

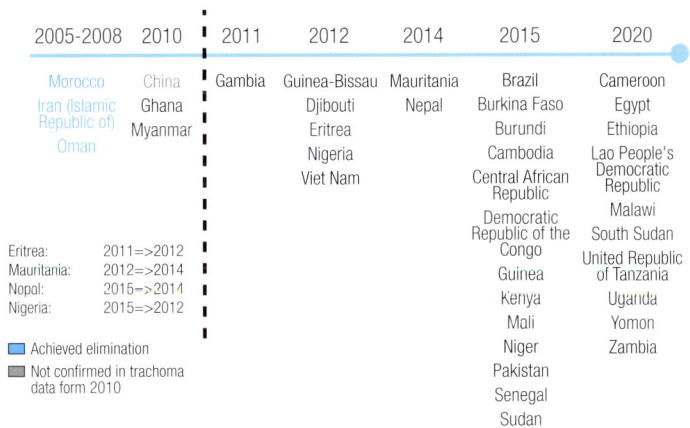

Fig. 5.3.2 Target dates set by Member States for eliminating blinding trachoma

Assessment

Implementation of the SAFE strategy should lead to the elimination of blinding trachoma (trichiasis) by 2020 in accordance with World Health Assembly resolution WHA51.11 adopted in 1998. Based on information reported to WHO, in 2008 about 60% of the population in need received preventive chemotherapy using antibiotics and about 45% received surgical care. The Islamic Republic of Iran, Morocco and Oman have reported reaching their elimination targets, but the global prevalence of blinding trachoma still must be reduced from the estimated 8 million cases of trichiasis (*3*).

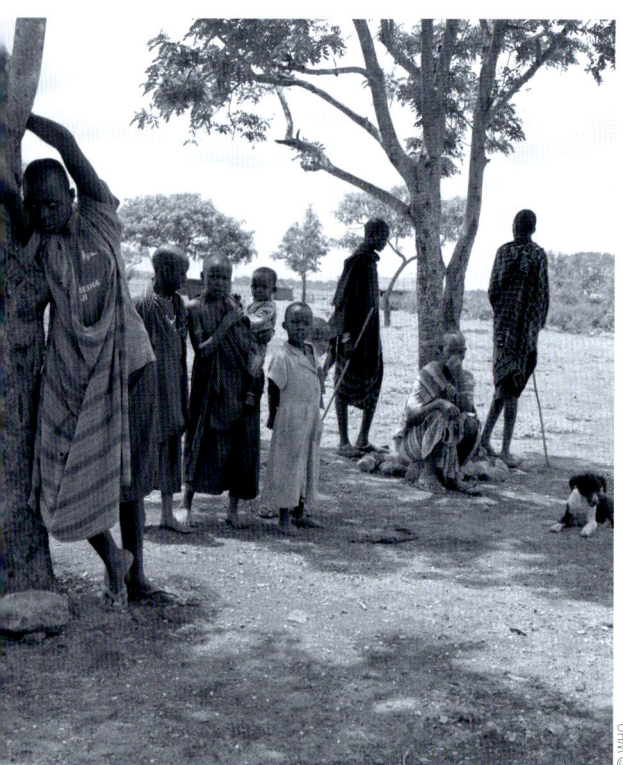

Masai village, United Republic of Tanzania. Despite surgery, Mzurisana (seen leaning against the tree) still cannot see well enough to make the necklaces that she once sold as her main source of income. She survives on the little money she earns by selling milk and borrowing food from neighbours. She cannot afford to send her children to school. Mzurisana's plight could have been prevented by better community education about eye health and more accessible health care services.

REFERENCES

1. Resnikoff S et al. Global magnitude of visual impairment caused by uncorrected refractive errors in 2004. *Bulletin of the World Health Organization*, 2008, 86:63–70.
2. Barenfanger J. Studies on the role of the family unit in the transmission of trachoma. *American Journal of Tropical Medicine and Hygiene*, 1975, 24:509–515.
3. Mariotti SP, Pascolini D, Rose-Nussbaumer J. Trachoma: global magnitude of a preventable cause of blindness. *British Journal of Ophthalmology*, 2009, 93:563–568.
4. Frick KD et al. Trichiasis and disability in a trachoma-endemic area of Tanzania. *Archives of Ophthalmology*, 2001, 119:1839–1844.
5. Kirkwood B et al. Relationships between mortality, visual acuity and microfilarial load in the area of the Onchocerciasis Control Programme. *Transactions of the Royal Society of Tropical Medicine and Hygiene*, 1983, 77:862–868.
6. Taylor HR et al. Increase in mortality associated with blindness in rural Africa. *Bulletin of the World Health Organization*, 1991, 69:335–338.
7. Bailey R et al. The duration of human ocular *Chlamydia trachomatis* infection is age dependent. *Epidemiology and Infection*, 1999, 123:479–486.
8. West SK et al. The epidemiology of trachoma in central Tanzania. *International Journal of Epidemiology*, 1991, 20:1088–1092.
9. Courtright P et al. Trachoma and blindness in the Nile Delta: current patterns and projections for the future in the rural Egyptian population. *British Journal of Ophthalmology*, 1989, 73:536–540.
10. Frick KD, Hanson CL, Jacobson GA. Global burden of trachoma and economics of the disease. *American Journal of Tropical Medicine and Hygiene*, 2003, 69:1–10.
11. *Global elimination of blinding trachoma (Resolution WHA51.11)*. [Adopted by the Fifty-first World Health Assembly on 16 May 1998.] Geneva, World Health Organization, 1998.
12. Sumamo E et al. The Cochrane library and trachoma: an overview of reviews. *Evidence-Based Child Health*, 2007, 2:943–964.
13. West ES et al. Risk factors for postsurgical trichiasis recurrence in a trachoma-endemic area. *Investigative Ophthalmology & Visual Science*, 2005, 46: 447–453.
14. Evans TG et al. Cost-effectiveness and cost utility of preventing tachomatous visual impairment: lessons from 30 years of trachoma control in Burma. *British Journal of Ophthalmology*, 1996, 80:880–889.
15. Baltussen RM et al. Cost-effectiveness of trachoma control in seven world regions. *Ophthalmic Epidemiology*, 2005, 12:91–101.

5.4 Buruli ulcer (*Mycobacterium ulcerans* infection)

Abstract

Buruli ulcer, a chronic necrotizing skin disease caused by infection with *Mycobacterium ulcerans*, has been reported to WHO from more than 33 countries. Globally, there is no clear trend in the number of cases, but an increasing trend has been found in Benin. Treatment is long and complicated unless early diagnosis is made. Buruli ulcer has been shown to have an annual economic impact per patient ranging from US$ 76 to US$ 428 in Ghana (*1*).

Description

The bacterium that causes Buruli ulcer belongs to the genus of bacteria that causes tuberculosis and leprosy. *Mycobacterium ulcerans* produces mycolactone, a toxin responsible for the extensive destruction of skin and soft tissue that leads to the formation of large ulcers, usually on the legs or arms. Most patients in Africa are children aged 14 years or younger (*2*). In endemic areas, clinical diagnosis is straightforward for experienced health-care workers. The four laboratory methods for confirming diagnosis, which depend on resources available locally and at national level, are (i) direct smear examination, for example, Ziehl Neelsen staining technique; (ii) polymerase-chain reaction; (iii) culture of *M. ulcerans*; and (iv) histopathology (*3*). Currently, WHO recommends (i) a combination of rifampicin and streptomycin or amikacin for 8 weeks; (ii) surgery to remove necrotic tissue, cover skin defects and correct deformities; and (iii) interventions to minimize or prevent disabilities (*4, 5*). Early detection and treatment of cases are essential in preventing disabilities. Patients who are not treated at an early stage of infection often suffer long-term functional disability, including restricted joint movement and visible cosmetic problems that produce negative social and economic impacts. The mode of transmission is under investigation, and there is no vaccine to prevent the disease.

Distribution and trends

Buruli ulcer has been reported in more than 33 countries, mainly in those with tropical and subtropical climates (*6*) (*Figure 5.4.1*). In 2009, cases were reported from about half of these countries, most of which are in Africa, where efforts to control the disease have been focused during the past decade. The data available to WHO are limited for three reasons: (i) within endemic countries where cases are being reported regularly, control activities are limited in geographical scope and the data may not therefore reflect the burden at the national level; (ii) there are large areas where limited or no activities are being carried out and the extent of the disease is therefore relatively unknown; (iii) limited knowledge of the disease, its focal distribution and the fact that it affects mainly poor rural communities all contribute to low reporting of cases.

Fig. 5.4.1 Distribution of Buruli ulcer, worldwide, 2008

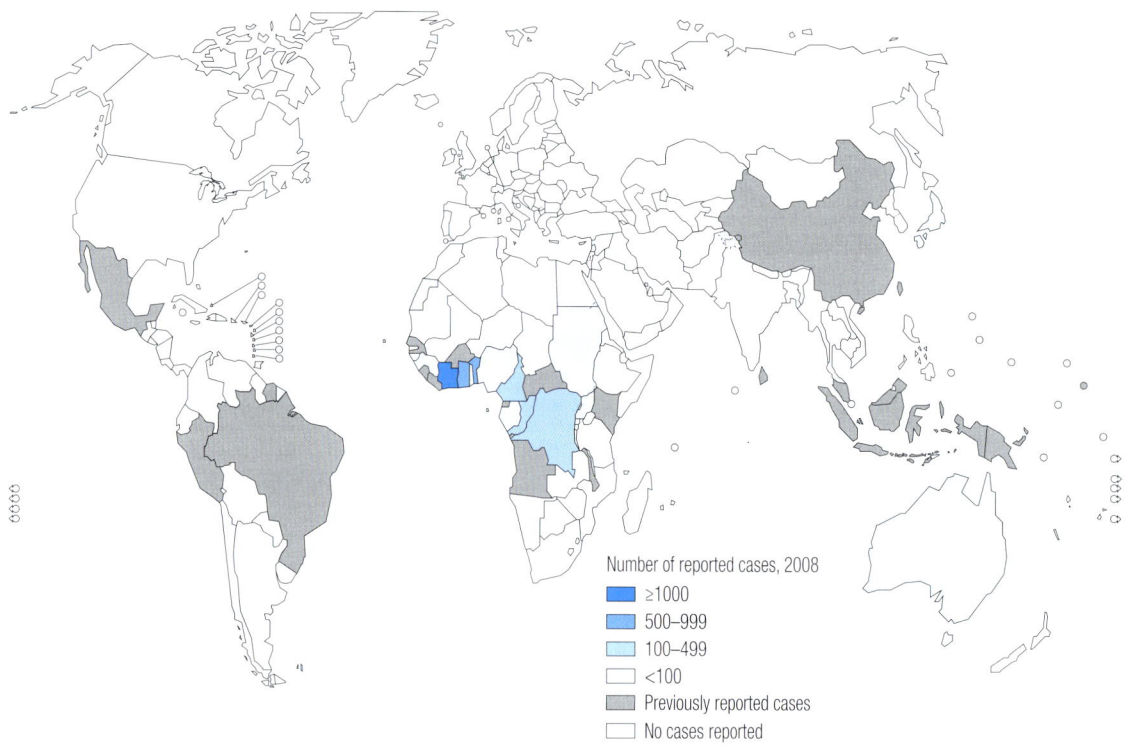

Globally, there is no clear trend in the number of cases reported to WHO (*Figure 5.4.2*). In certain communities and countries, obvious trends of increasing numbers have occurred during the past decade. There has been an increasing trend in the number of cases in Benin since 1989, when the first cases were reported (*Figure 5.4.3*).

Fig. 5.4.2 Number of new cases of Buruli ulcer reported to WHO, worldwide, 2004–2009

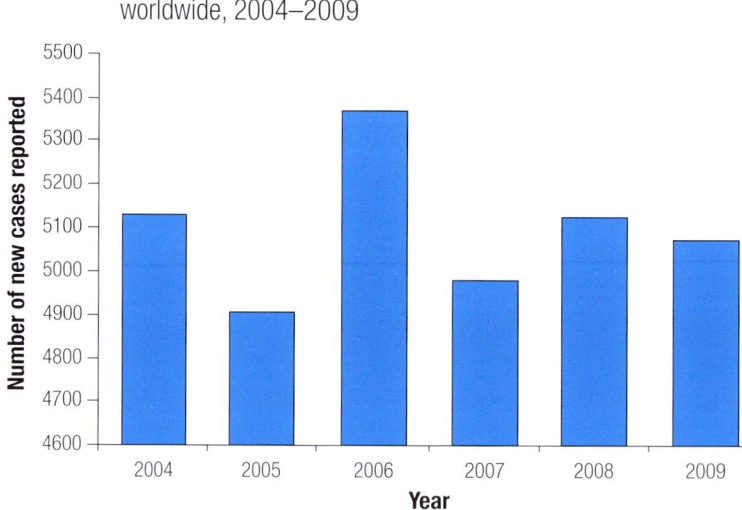

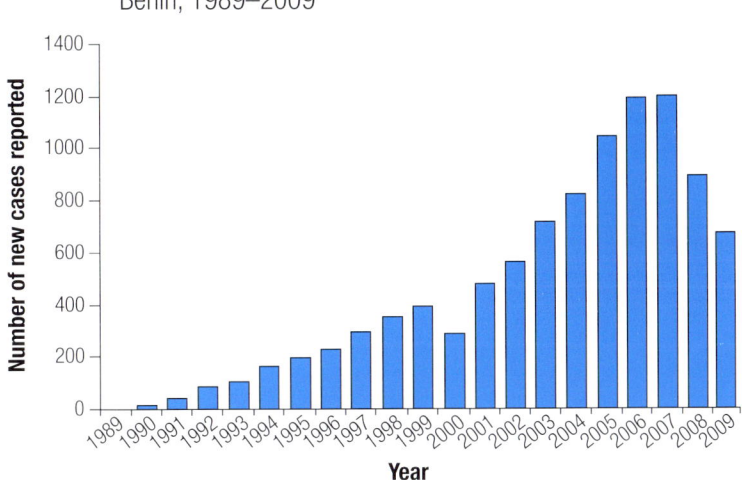

Fig. 5.4.3 Number of new cases of Buruli ulcer reported to WHO, Benin, 1989–2009

Morbidity

The main problems caused by Buruli ulcer are the long periods needed for healing, which include hospitalization, and contractures resulting from healing in late disease, especially when lesions cross joints and treatment is inadequate. Some studies have estimated that about 25% of healed cases have some extent of disability (*7*). Other studies have arrived at higher percentages, depending on the extent of early-detection activities taking place in the study area – that is, if there are fewer detection activities then the proportion of those who become disabled will be higher. About 55% of cases occur in children, and there is no difference between males and females as far as the frequency of infection is concerned (*8*). The few cases of death in patients are related to secondary causes (sepsis and tetanus).

Economic impact

Buruli ulcer imposes an economic burden on affected households and on health systems that are involved in diagnosis and treatment. In Ghana during 2001–2003, the median annual total cost of the disease to a household, by stage of disease, ranged from US$ 76.20 (16% of a work year) per patient with a lesion to US$ 428 (89% of a work year) per patient who had undergone amputation (*9*). The average cost of treating a case was estimated to be US$ 780 per patient during 1994–1996, an amount that far exceeded per capita government spending on health (*7*). In Australia during 1997–1998, the average cost of diagnosing Buruli ulcer and treating a patient was AUS$ 14 608 (*10*), an amount approximately seven times greater than the average national health expenditure per person (AUS$ 2557). In a study conducted in 2008 in Cameroon (*11*), hospitalization costs accounted for 25% of households' yearly earnings; median total costs of hospital treatment were €126.70. In addition to preventing disabilities, early detection and treatment of cases are therefore economical and should be widely promoted.

Prevention and control

In many countries, activities to control the disease through early case-detection and treatment are restricted by limited resources. Treatment facilities are limited in affected areas, but the move towards decentralized delivery of antibiotic therapy should increase coverage. The cost of interventions includes that for implementing early detection and health education efforts at the community level, training health workers, providing rifampicin and streptomycin, supporting surgical treatment for complicated cases, and rehabilitating those with deformities.

Assessment

Resolution WHA57.1 adopted by the World Health Assembly in 2004 urges endemic countries to intensify control activities and accelerate research. The priority is to improve early detection and case-management in the absence of a vaccine. Basic research is needed to understand the biology and epidemiology of the causative agent of this emerging disease.

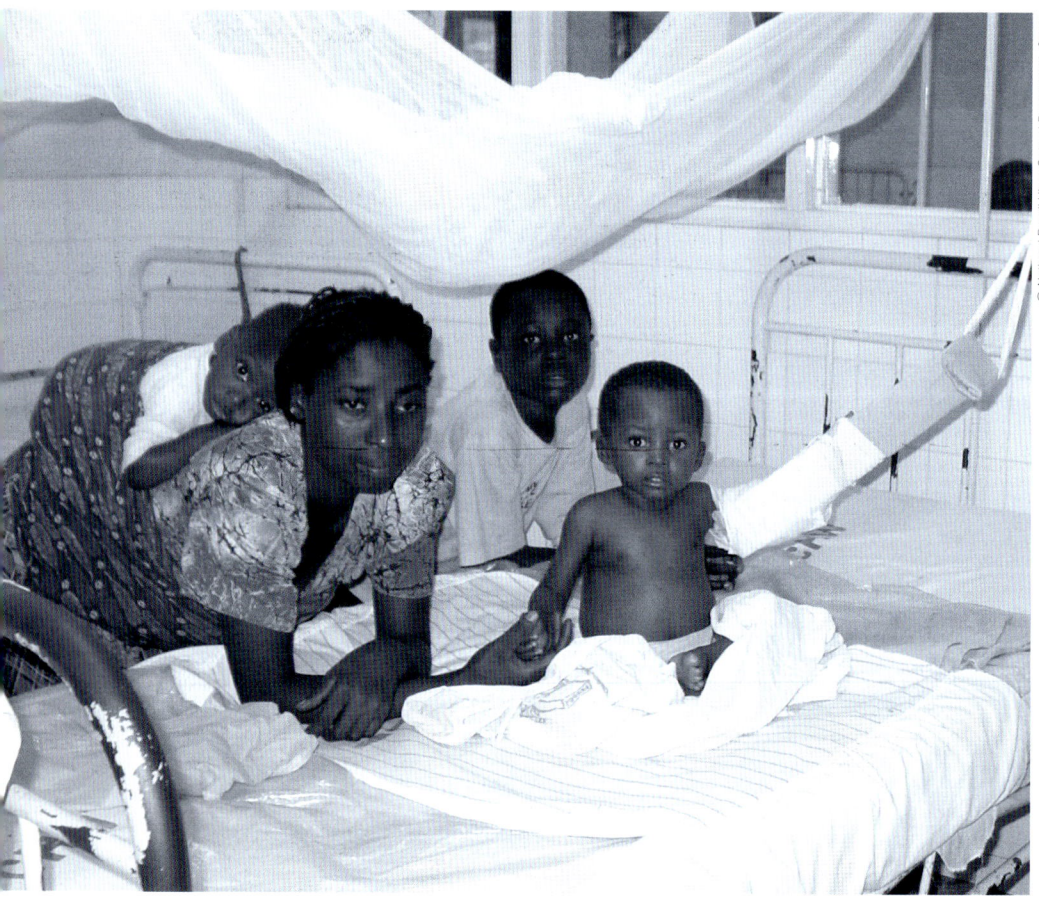

Child receiving treatment at Agogo hospital, Ghana. Early detection of Buruli ulcer disease is crucial to prevent complications and surgery.

REFERENCES

1. *Abstracts of the annual meeting on Buruli ulcer, 14–17 March 2005*. Geneva, World Health Organization, 2006.

2. Asiedu K, Sherpbier R, Raviglione M, eds. *Buruli ulcer: Mycobacterium ulcerans infection*. Geneva, World Health Organization Global Buruli Ulcer Initiative, 2000 (WHO/CDS/CPE/GBUI/200.1).

3. Portaels F, Johnson P, Meyers WM, eds. *Buruli ulcer. Diagnosis of Mycobacterium ulcerans disease: a manual for health care providers*. Geneva, World Health Organization, 2000.

4. *Provisional guidance on the role of specific antibiotics in the management of Mycobacterium ulcerans disease (Buruli ulcer)*. Geneva, World Health Organization, 2004 (WHO/CDS/CPE/GBUI.10, 2004).

5. Nienhuis WA et al. Antimicrobial treatment for early, limited *Mycobacterium ulcerans* infection: a randomised controlled trial. *Lancet*, 2010 (published online 4 February 2010).

6. Buruli ulcer disease – *Mycobacterium ulcerans* infection: an overview of reported cases globally. *Weekly Epidemiological Record*, 2004, 79: 194–199.

7. Asiedu K, Etuaful SA. Socioeconomic implications of Buruli ulcer in Ghana: a three-year review. *American Journal of Tropical Medicine and Hygiene*, 1998, 59:1015–1022.

8. Sopoh GE et al. Buruli ulcer surveillance, Benin, 2003–2005. *Emerging Infectious Diseases*, 2007, 13:1374–1376.

9. *Economic burden of Buruli ulcer on households in the Central and Ashanti regions of Ghana. Report of the 7th WHO Advisory Group Meeting on Buruli ulcer, 8–11 March 2004*. Geneva, World Health Organization, 2004 (WHO/CDS/CPE/GBUI/2004.9).

10. Drummond C, Butler JRG. *Mycobacterium ulcerans* treatment costs, self-reported data, Australia. *Emerging Infectious Diseases*, 2004, 10:1038–1043.

11. Peeters Grietens K et al. "It is me who endures but my family that suffers": social isolation as a consequence of the household cost burden of Buruli ulcer free of charge hospital treatment. *PLoS Neglected Tropical Diseases*, 2008, 2(10):e321.

5.5 Endemic treponematoses

Abstract

Endemic treponematoses, which comprise yaws, endemic syphilis (bejel) and pinta, are caused by bacteria of the genus *Treponema*. By the early 1970s, prevalence of the diseases had been reduced from 50 million to 2.5 million cases following the widespread use of long-lasting injectable penicillin. This progress was not maintained.

Description

The endemic treponematoses are a group of chronic bacterial infections caused by treponemes (*1*). Yaws is caused by *Treponema pallidum pertenue*, endemic syphilis by *T. pallidum endemicum*, and pinta by *T. pallidum carateum*. These organisms are morphologically and serologically indistinguishable from the organism that causes venereal syphilis (*T. pallidum pallidum*). Yaws is the most prevalent disease. Endemic treponematoses cause disfigurement and disability if left untreated. One of the major success stories in public health was the treatment campaign led by WHO and UNICEF in the 1950s and 1960s, which reached 50 million individuals in 46 countries, and reduced the global burden of the endemic treponematoses to 2.5 million cases by the end of the campaigns in the early 1970s (*2*, *3*). Penicillin was responsible for this achievement. The absence of continued surveillance in the remaining endemic countries allowed treponematoses to persist; their resurgence in the late 1970s led to the adoption by the World Health Assembly of resolution WHA31.58 in 1978, which aimed to implement integrated treponematoses control programmes and place particular emphasis on active surveillance to interrupt transmission of the diseases at the earliest possible time in the areas where they are endemic and to prevent their recurrence in areas from which they have been eliminated or where they have never been endemic. This was followed by renewed control efforts in west Africa in the early 1980s, but these were not sustained.

Yaws and endemic syphilis affect the skin and bone, while pinta is confined to the skin. Poor personal hygiene and overcrowding facilitate their spread. Clinical manifestations are modified by climate, season and the level of endemicity in the affected geographical area. Diagnosis often relies on clinical findings. Serological tests available for diagnosis are: the rapid plasmin reagin test, the venereal disease research laboratory nontreponemal test, the treponemal pallidum haemagglutination assay and the fluorescent treponemal antibody absorption test. The results from these tests are helpful but should be interpreted in the context of clinical findings, the age of the patient and the endemicity of the area.

Distribution

The global extent of endemic treponematoses remains unknown. Treponematoses have been largely eliminated or significantly reduced in many of the 46 countries that were endemic in the 1950s. Relatively few countries were endemic for these diseases in the 1990s; their status in 2008 is shown in *Figure 5.5.1*. The last estimate by WHO in 1995 yielded a global prevalence of 2.5 million cases, of which 460 000 were considered infectious (3). Most cases were in the African Region. Since the early 1990s, there has been no formal reporting of cases to WHO, and programmes to control these diseases have largely disappeared. Only five countries maintain some activities to control yaws. Since 2004, India has reported zero cases after intense efforts to eliminate the disease (4). Indonesia, while remaining the major endemic area in the South-East Asia Region, still maintains its control programme (5). Papua New Guinea occasionally reports data through the routine surveillance system and remains the major endemic area in the Western Pacific Region.

Fig. 5.5.1 Distribution of endemic treponematoses, worldwide, 2008

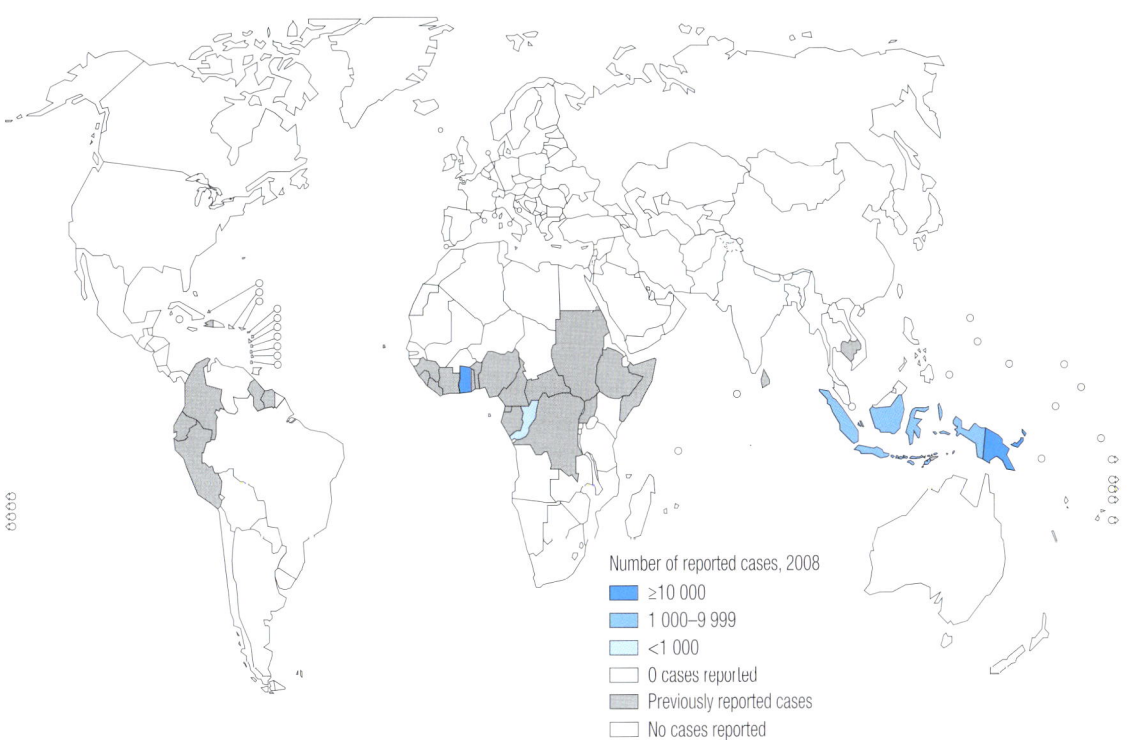

Ghana has a significant number of yaws cases and maintains its control programme. In Congo, cases of yaws occur among the pygmy population in the regions of Likouala, Lekoumou and Sangha, and a survey in 2009 identified 646

clinical cases (6). In 2008, a survey carried out in Lomie Health District in the Eastern province of Cameroon identified 167 clinical cases among the pygmy population (personal communication, national coordinator for Leprosy, Buruli ulcer and yaws, 2009). Cases have been reported in Côte d'Ivoire (7) and the Democratic Republic of the Congo (8).

There are no clear patterns in the number of cases reported, such as that seen in the obvious trend in Indonesia (*Figure 5.5.2*). As renewed interest increases and activities intensify in affected countries as part of NTD control programmes, the full extent of endemic treponematoses, including trends over time, should become apparent.

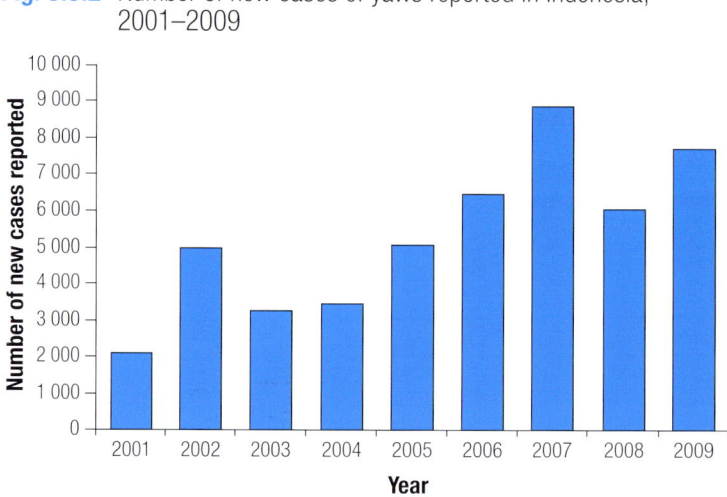

Fig. 5.5.2 Number of new cases of yaws reported in Indonesia, 2001–2009

Morbidity

Ulcerative cases may become infected and can lead to severe secondary bacterial infection including tetanus. Long-term complications of yaws (arising 5 or more years later) occur in 10% of untreated cases, leading to disfigurement of the face and legs. Yaws most frequently affects children, and infection peaks in those aged 2–10 years (9). Of new cases, 75% occur in children younger than 14 years. For pinta, the age range is 10–30 years. Yaws affects boys more often than girls; in endemic syphilis and pinta there is no difference between males and females in the number affected.

There are no estimates of the economic impact of endemic treponematoses. Since these diseases respond well to penicillin, it is unlikely that their long-term economic impact would be considerable, although a few cases of disfiguring complications may have a social rather than an economic impact. Motivation for action against endemic treponematoses is based on humanitarian reasons: since effective and inexpensive treatment is available, the persistence of treponematoses is medically and socially unacceptable. There is no reported mortality associated with endemic treponematoses.

Prevention and control

Control and treatment policies developed primarily for yaws decades ago are still applicable for all the endemic treponematoses today: where prevalence is more than 10%, the entire population should be treated; where prevalence is 5–10%, all active cases, children aged younger than 14 years and obvious contacts should be treated; where prevalence is less than 5%, all active cases, household members and obvious contacts should be treated. Treatment of these infections involves a single injection of long-acting benzathine penicillin. The recommended single doses are 600 000 units for children younger than 6 years, 1.2 million units for those aged 6–14 years and 2.4 million units for those older than 14 years (*1*).

In 2007, WHO launched a renewed attempt to eliminate yaws and related diseases with a strategy for their control and eventual elimination based on four components: (i) identification of the population at risk of infection; (ii) case-finding (active and passive); (iii) treatment of cases and contacts; and (iv) surveillance (using standardized recording and reporting systems) (*2*).

Assessment

Complete interruption of transmission as envisaged by resolution WHA31.58 adopted in 1978 has not been attained because the control programmes stopped. Renewal of prevention and control activities requires active case-finding and improved treatment, preferably using non-injectable antibiotics (*10–12*).

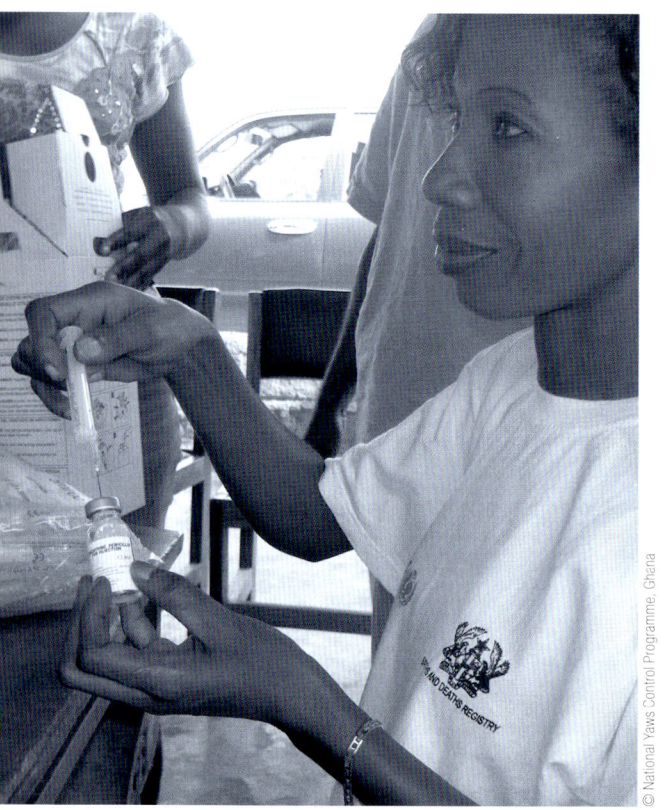

Health care worker preparing benzathine penicillin in a yaws treatment campaign, West Akim district, Ghana.

Yaws is cured by a single dose of benzathine penicillin which can prevent chronic disfigurement and disability.

REFERENCES

1. Perine PL et al. *Handbook of endemic treponematoses: yaws, endemic syphilis and pinta*. Geneva, World Health Organization, 1984.
2. *Yaws*. Geneva, World Health Organization, 2010.
3. *Informal consultation on endemic treponematoses, 6–7 July 1995*. Geneva, World Health Organization, 1995 (WHO/EMC/95.3).
4. Elimination of yaws in India. *Weekly Epidemiological Record*, 2008, 83:125–132.
5. *Strategy for yaws eradication in the South-East Asia Region*. New Delhi, World Health Organization, Regional Office for South-East Asia, 2010.
6. Obvala D. Activities to control endemic treponematoses in the Congo [abstract]. In: *Report of the annual meeting on Buruli ulcer, 31 March–2 April 2009, Cotonou, Benin*. Geneva, World Health Organization, 2009.
7. Touré B et al. Le Pian en Côte d'Ivoire : problème de santé oublié et négligé [Yaws in Côte d'Ivoire: a health problem forgotten and neglected]. *Bulletin de la Société de Pathologie Exotique*, 2007, 100(2):130–132.
8. Gerstl S et al. Prevalence study of yaws in the Democratic Republic of Congo using the lot quality assurance sampling method. *PLoS ONE*, 2009, 4(7):e6338.
9. Meheus AZ, Narain JP, Asiedu KB. Endemic treponematoses. In: Cohen J, Powderly SM, Opal WG, eds. *Infectious diseases*, 3rd ed. London, Elsevier, 2010 [in press (Chapter 105)].
10. *International Task Force for Disease Eradication: summary of the eleventh meeting of the ITFDE (II)*. Atlanta, GA, The Carter Center, 2007.
11. Asiedu K. The return of yaws. *Bulletin of the World Health Organization*, 2008, 86:507–508.
12. Rinaldi A. Yaws: a second (and maybe last?) chance for eradication. *PLoS Neglected Tropical Diseases*, 2008, 2(8):e275.

5.6 Leprosy (Hansen disease)

Abstract

Of 122 countries considered to be endemic for leprosy, 119 have eliminated the disease as a public-health problem (defined as achieving a prevalence of less than 1 case/10 000 population). The 213 000 cases reported are confined mostly to 17 countries reporting more than 1000 cases annually. This figure reflects a reduction of more than 90% in the number of cases detected globally since 1985, mainly as a result of timely case-finding and multidrug therapy, which have also prevented disabilities caused by leprosy in 1–2 million people. Transmission of the bacterium (*Mycobacterium leprae*) continues in limited geographical areas in several countries that have reached the national elimination target.

Description

Leprosy results from a slowly progressive bacterial infection with *Mycobacterium leprae*. The disease mainly affects the skin, peripheral nerves, lining of the upper respiratory tract, eyes and other organs. Leprosy affects people of all ages and both sexes. The standard treatment for leprosy – multidrug therapy (a combination of rifampicin, dapsone and clofazimine) – was recommended in 1981 by a WHO Study Group on chemotherapy for leprosy (*1*). Multidrug therapy, which replaced dapsone monotherapy, prevents the development of disabilities by providing an early cure, and it prevents the emergence of drug resistance (*2*). Left untreated, leprosy causes permanent damage to the skin, nerves, limbs and eyes. For centuries, people suffering from leprosy were subject to discrimination, stigmatization and exclusion.

Leprosy is not highly infectious because most people have natural immunity. In addition, once patients start multidrug therapy they are no longer infectious. The exact mode of transmission is not known but probably occurs through droplets from the nose and mouth during close and frequent contact with untreated cases. Diagnosis commonly relies on clinical signs and symptoms. Only in rare instances are laboratory and other investigations needed to confirm a diagnosis.

Distribution and trends

Since 1985, the reported prevalence of leprosy has been reduced by more than 90%, and more than 15 million patients have been cured (*Figure 5.6.1*). To date, 119/122 countries considered to be endemic for leprosy have eliminated the disease as a public-health problem (*Table 5.6.1*).

Fig. 5.6.1 Leprosy prevalence rates, data reported to WHO as of January 2009

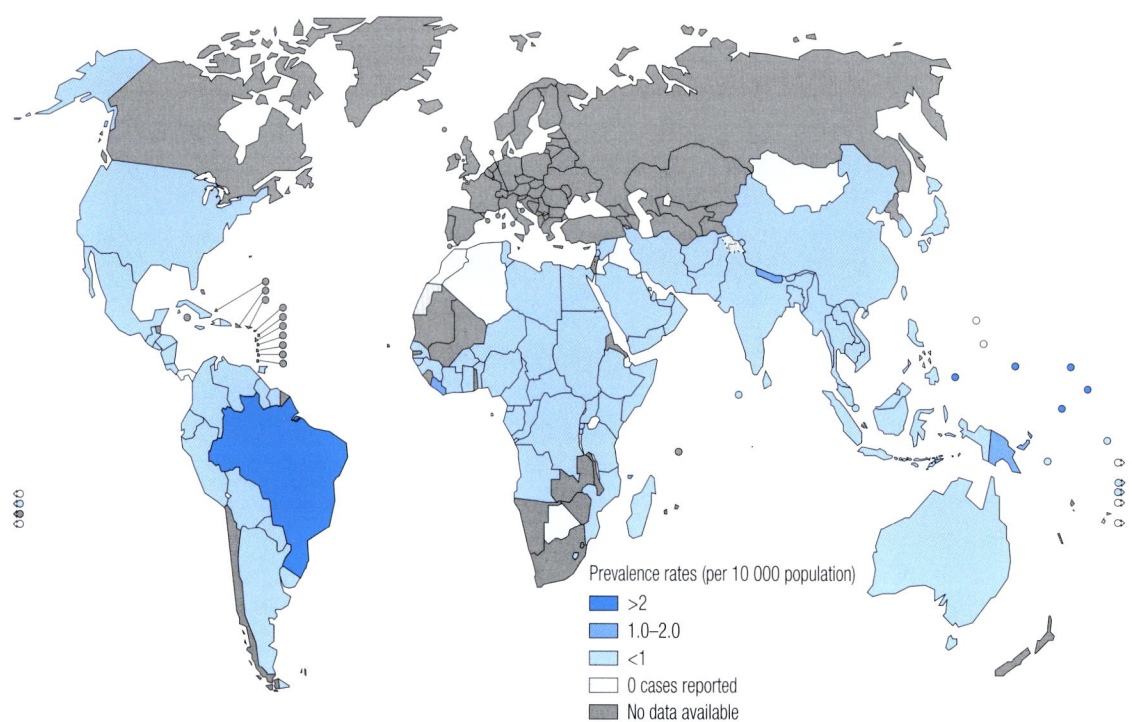

In 2009, a total of 121 countries or territories reported on leprosy to WHO: 31 from the African Region, 25 from the Region of the Americas, 10 from the South-East Asia Region, 22 from the Eastern Mediterranean Region and 33 from the Western Pacific Region. At the beginning of 2009, there were 213 036 cases registered globally (*3*).

Table 5.6.1 Trends in the detection of new leprosy cases, by WHO region (excluding the European Region), 2002–2008 (*3*)

WHO region	Number of new cases detected annually						
	2002	2003	2004	2005	2006	2007	2008
African	48 248	47 006	46 918	45 179	34 480	34 468	29 814
Americas	39 939	52 435	52 662	41 952	47 612	42 135	41 891
South-East Asia	520 632	405 147	298 603	201 635	174 118	171 576	167 505
Eastern Mediterranean	4 665	3 940	3 392	3 133	3 261	4 091	3 938
Western Pacific	7 154	6 190	6 216	7 137	6 190	5 863	5 859
Total	620 638	514 718	407 791	299 036	265 661	258 133	249 007

During 2008, only 17 countries reported more than 1000 new cases, accounting for 94% of the new cases detected globally.

Variations exist among countries in all regions in the proportion of newly detected cases of multibacillary disease among children and women, and of those with grade-two disabilities. In the African Region, the proportion of cases with multibacillary disease ranges from 20% in Cameroon to 92% in Kenya. In the Region of the Americas, the proportion ranges from 39% in the Plurinational State of Bolivia to 78% in Mexico. In the South-East Asia Region, the proportion ranges from 45% in Bangladesh to 82% in Indonesia. In the Eastern Mediterranean Region, the proportion ranges from 30% in Somalia to 89% in Egypt. In the Western Pacific Region, the Federated States of Micronesia reported that 58% of newly detected cases had multibacillary disease; the Philippines reported 90%.

Trends in the number of newly detected cases (*Table 5.6.1*) mirror the implementation or phasing out of major operational activities (*Table 5.6.2*). During 1991–1995, the number of new cases reflected the absence of major control efforts: new cases were detected by passive case detection and were typically treated with dapsone monotherapy. In the mid-1990s, the availability of free multidrug therapy gave new impetus to control efforts. Leprosy elimination campaigns and special action programmes for leprosy elimination were carried out to detect cases and treat patients with multidrug therapy. These campaigns relied on strong community mobilization to dispel the stigma associated with leprosy, and encouraged hidden cases to seek treatment; hence, the large increase in new cases, peaking at 804 367 in 1998. The new-case detection rate remained high until 2001 as the backlog of cases was detected and treated. Many endemic countries have fully integrated leprosy control into their primary health-care system. From 2002, active case-finding was scaled back, and from 2005 onwards the number of new cases has remained static at about 250 000 cases annually (*Figure 5.6.2*).

Table 5.6.2 Key stages in leprosy control and elimination

Phase	Years	Activity	Impact
Phase I	1982–1986	Introduction of multidrug therapy on a pilot basis in some countries; updating of leprosy registers to reflect actual numbers	Reduction in prevalence
Phase II	1987–1994	Steady increase in coverage of multidrug therapy	Prevalence further reduced due to cure of patients
Phase III	1995–2000	Dramatic increase in coverage of multidrug therapy with the provision of free multidrug therapy through WHO; large-scale communication campaigns to destigmatize leprosy and promote active case-finding activities	Large increase in number of new cases detected
Phase IV	2000–2003	Continued availability of free multidrug therapy; updating of multidrug therapy registers and activities to address operational problems; targeted leprosy elimination campaigns implemented in highly endemic areas	Decreasing prevalence and decreasing case detection
Phase V	2003–2009	Sustained implementation of multidrug therapy and passive case detection	Steady reduction in case detection and prevalence

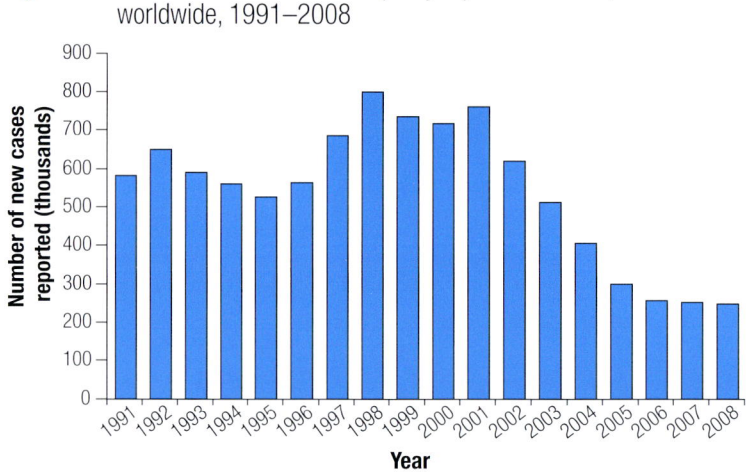

Fig. 5.6.2 Number of new cases of leprosy reported to WHO, worldwide, 1991–2008

The South-East Asia Region continues to report most of the world's leprosy cases (*Figure 5.6.3*).

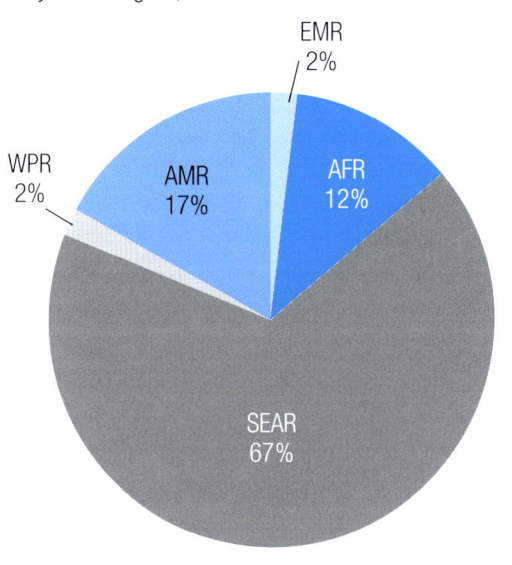

Fig. 5.6.3 Distribution of new cases of leprosy reported to WHO, by WHO region, 2008

AFR – African / AMR – The Americas / EMR – Eastern Mediterranean / SEAR – South-East Asia / WPR – Western Pacific

In most countries, leprosy is more often diagnosed in men than in women. It is not clear whether the higher leprosy rates in men reflect epidemiological differences or the influence of operational factors (*4*). Timely case-finding and delivery of multidrug therapy have prevented disabilities caused by leprosy among an estimated 1–2 million people (*5*).

Economic impact

Costs associated with control include those of case detection, treatment, prevention of disability and rehabilitation. As case-detection rates decrease, the average cost of detecting a case increases. Many leprosy control programmes now rely on voluntary case-finding supported by information, education and communication activities to raise and maintain awareness of the early signs and symptoms of leprosy. Costs of diagnosis and treatment have fallen steadily, and diagnosis by clinical examination only is now recommended. The average cost of finding, treating, preventing disability in and rehabilitating a new case ranges from US$ 76 to US$ 264 (*6*). The cost per DALY of detecting and treating a new case of leprosy is estimated to be US$ 38; for patients needing treatment for reactions and ulcers the cost per DALY is estimated to be US$ 7; for those needing footwear and self-care education the cost is estimated at US$ 75; and for those requiring reconstructive surgery it is US$ 110.

Data on the economic effect of leprosy at the national level are not available, but leprosy affects the economically active, and the incidence peaks among those aged 10–20 years and 30–50 years. Studies of the impact of leprosy on productivity show that deformity from leprosy reduces the chances of obtaining employment and reduces household income and expenditure on food (*7, 8*).

Prevention and control

The dramatic impact of multidrug therapy led to the adoption in 1991 by the World Health Assembly of resolution WHA44.9 to eliminate leprosy as a public-health problem by 2000. Elimination is defined as reducing the prevalence of the disease to less than 1 case/10 000 people. The strategy to eliminate leprosy as a public-health problem has two elements: (i) improving access to early diagnosis by integrating leprosy control services into existing public-health services; and (ii) providing free multidrug therapy. The early detection of cases has reduced the risk of deformities and disabilities, ensuring that people affected by leprosy can lead normal lives with dignity.

The scaling up of access to multidrug therapy took place during several distinct phases (*Table 5.6.2*). The slow uptake in the first two phases was due to the higher cost of multidrug therapy compared with dapsone monotherapy. Additionally, staff providing leprosy control services needed to be retrained and reorganized to provide monthly treatment instead of the earlier regimen of lifelong treatment provided annually. The provision of free multidrug therapy for all patients was the turning point in the effort against leprosy. With assured supplies of multidrug therapy, health ministries in endemic countries scaled up access to diagnosis and treatment.

Assessment

Early case detection and multidrug therapy will remain the key elements of the leprosy-control strategy in the foreseeable future. There is a need to maintain the free supply of medicines used for multidrug therapy. The goal of eliminating leprosy as a public-health problem has been shown to be attainable. Resource-constrained countries have achieved that goal.

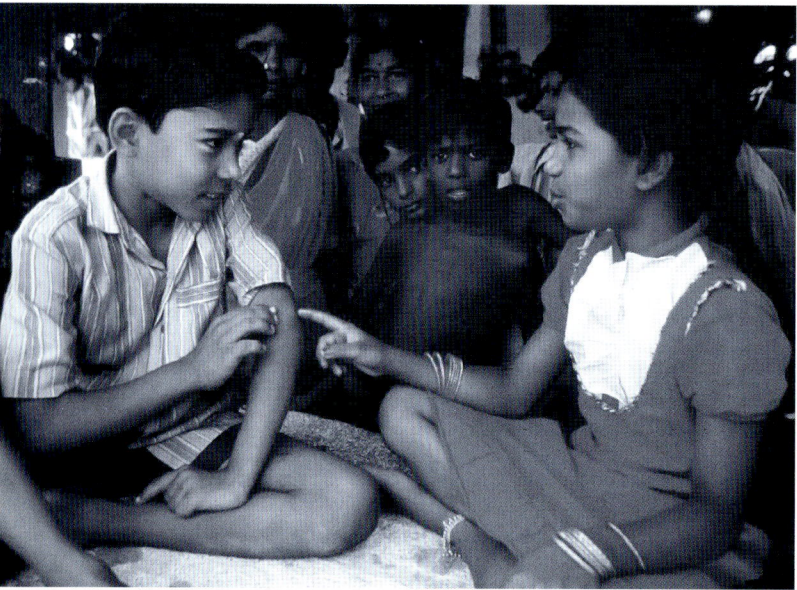

Students discussing leprosy at school in India. Access to information, diagnosis and treatment with multidrug therapy (MDT) remain key elements of WHO's drive to eliminate leprosy.

REFERENCES

1. *Chemotherapy of leprosy for control programmes: report of a WHO Study Group.* Geneva, World Health Organization, 1982 (WHO Technical Report Series, No. 675).
2. *Risk of relapse in leprosy.* Geneva, World Health Organization, 1994 (WHO/CTD/LEP/94.1).
3. Leprosy: global situation. *Weekly Epidemiological Record*, 2009, 84:333–340.
4. Doull J A et al. The incidence of leprosy in Cordova and Talisay, Cebu, Philippines. *International Journal of Leprosy*, 1942, 10:107–131.
5. Leprosy disabilities: magnitude of the problem. *Weekly Epidemiological Record*, 1995, 70:269–275.
6. Jan HF et al. Tropical diseases targeted for elimination: Chagas disease, lymphatic filariasis, onchocerciasis, and leprosy. In: Jamison DT et al., eds. *Disease control priorities in developing countries*, 2nd ed. New York, Oxford University Press, 2006:433–450.
7. Diffey B et al. The effect of leprosy-induced deformity on the nutritional status of index cases and their household members in rural South India: a socioeconomic perspective. *European Journal of Clinical Nutrition*, 2000, 54(8):643–649.
8. Kopparty SN. Problems, acceptance, and social inequality: a study of the deformed leprosy patients and their families. *Leprosy Review*, 1995, 66(3):239–249.

5.7 Chagas disease (American trypanosomiasis)

Abstract

Chagas disease continues to persist in the Region of the Americas, but the estimated number of infected people has fallen from approximately 20 million in 1981 to around 10 million in 2009. The risk of transmission has been reduced by introducing vector-control measures and safer blood transfusions in Latin America. Population mobility has carried the disease to regions where the disease was previously unknown.

Description

Chagas disease is caused by the protozoan parasite *Trypanosoma cruzi*. Infection mainly occurs through contact with the faeces of a triatomine bug, which defecates after sucking blood at night. The insect resides in crevices in the walls and roofs of poorly constructed houses, usually in rural and periurban areas throughout Latin America. The parasite is transmitted when a person inadvertently enables the parasite-contaminated faeces to make contact with any break in the skin (including the bite), the eyes or mouth (*1*). Other modes of transmission include transfusion of infected blood (*2*), oral transmission through contaminated food (*3*), vertical transmission (*4*) and organ transplantation (*5*). Up to 30% of patients will develop heart damage, and up to 10% will develop damage to their oesophagus, colon or autonomic nervous system, or all of these, in the late chronic phase of the disease. Patients ultimately die, usually from sudden death caused by arrhythmias; this often occurs in early adulthood.

Distribution

About 10 million people worldwide are estimated to be infected with *T. cruzi*, mostly in the endemic areas of 21 Latin American countries: Argentina, Belize, the Bolivarian Republic of Venezuela, Brazil, Chile, Colombia, Costa Rica, Ecuador, El Salvador, French Guyana, Guatemala, Guyana, Honduras, Mexico, Nicaragua, Panama, Paraguay, Peru, the Plurinational State of Bolivia, Suriname and Uruguay (*6*) (*Figure 5.7.1*).

Fig. 5.7.1 Distribution of cases of *Trypanosoma cruzi* infection, based on official estimates and status of vector transmission, worldwide, 2006–2009

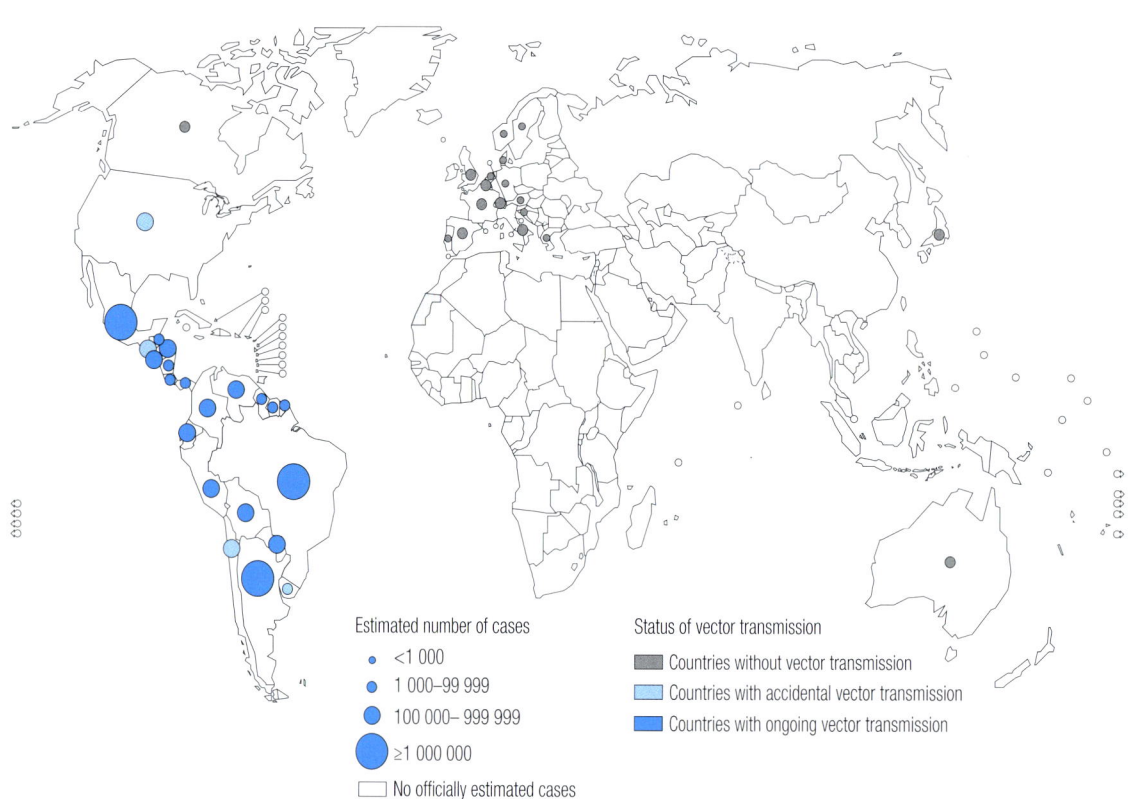

For thousands of years, Chagas disease was known only in the Region of the Americas, mainly in Latin America, where it has been endemic (*7*). In past decades, it has been increasingly detected in other non-endemic countries in the Region of the Americas (Canada and the United States of America), the Western Pacific Region (mainly Australia and Japan) and the European Region (mainly in Belgium, France, Italy, Spain, Switzerland and the United Kingdom, but also in Austria, Croatia, Denmark, Germany, Luxembourg, the Netherlands, Norway, Portugal, Romania and Sweden). The presence of Chagas disease outside Latin America is the result of population mobility, notably migration, but cases have been reported among travellers returning from Latin America and even in adopted children (*8*). Subsequent transmission occurs through transfusion or vertical and transplantation routes (*9*).

Morbidity

Chagas disease manifests in two phases. Initially, there is an acute phase, lasting for about 2 months, with a high parasitaemia in the blood. Most cases are asymptomatic or present nonspecific symptoms but, depending on the entrance point of the parasite into the body, the first sign can be a skin lesion (chagoma) or purplish swelling of one eyelid (Romaña sign) with locally enlarged lymph glands and fever lasting for several weeks. Other symptoms may include headache, pallor, muscle pain, difficulty in breathing, swelling of the legs or face, abdominal pain, cough, liver enlargement, rash, painful nodules, spleen enlargement, generalized body swelling, diarrhoea, multiple swollen lymph glands, heart inflammation (with chest pain and even heart failure) and, less frequently, meningoencephalitis (with seizures and even paralysis). The disease may be more severe in children younger than 2 years, the elderly, the immunosuppressed or in individuals infected with a high number of parasites, such as seen in foodborne outbreaks (oral transmission). In people with AIDS, meningoencephalitis is the most frequent manifestation.

The acute phase is followed by the chronic phase, with parasites hidden in target tissues, especially in the heart and digestive muscles. During this phase, different clinical forms may be observed: (i) the indeterminate or asymptomatic form – the most frequent form – is typically found immediately after the acute phase and is lifelong in most patients; (ii) the cardiac form occurs in up to 30% of the patients, with disorders of the heart's electrical conduction system, arrhythmia, heart-muscle disorder, heart failure and embolisms; (iii) the form of digestive lesions (enlargement of the oesophagus and the colon) has been observed south of the Amazon basin; and (iv) a mixed form (cardiac plus digestive) that affects up to 10% of patients (*10*). More than 10 000 deaths are estimated to occur annually from Chagas disease.

In areas with domiciliary vector transmission, typically children younger than 5 years are infected. In areas without domiciliary transmission, the infection is detected at older ages, and is usually related to agricultural, fishing or hunting activities that provide greater exposure to wildlife vectors. In general, there is no gender predominance in Chagas disease, but local variations exist depending on exposure to different routes of transmission. The incapacitating effects and mortality of Chagas disease have been one of the biggest public-health problems in Latin America. According to a published study (*11*), the 10-year mortality rate may range from 9% to 85%, depending on the cardiac damage.

Economic impact

The cost of treating Chagas disease is substantial, even though many people are not receiving appropriate care. A recent study (*12*) in Colombia estimated an average expected annual cost per patient with chronic Chagas disease of US$ 1028. On average, the estimated lifetime cost of treating a patient with chronic Chagas disease in Colombia is US$ 11 619. Without taking into account the number of infected patients who have not developed chronic alterations (these patients are also a burden on the health-care system), the same study calculated that the economic burden of the medical care of all patients who developed chronic conditions would be around US$ 267 million per year. Taking into account the dwellings that should be prioritized because of the risk of vector transmission, spraying activities would cost nearly US$ 5 million, or around 2% of the expected annual expenditure on health care. These rough estimations seem to confirm the potential of accruing not only economic savings but also, more importantly, avoiding disability and suffering.

Prevention and control

There have been national and international successes in parasite and vector control as a result of the Southern Cone Initiative, the Central American Initiative, the Andean Pact Initiative and the Amazonian Initiative, all of which were technically supported by the Pan American Health Organization. These multinational initiatives have led to substantial reductions in transmission by *Triatoma infestans*, the principal vector in the Southern Cone countries (Argentina, Brazil, Chile, Paraguay, the Plurinational State of Bolivia and Uruguay), and by *Rhodnius prolixus* in Central America. In addition, the risk of transmission by blood transfusion has been substantially reduced throughout Latin America. These advances have been achieved because of the commitment from Member States where the disease is endemic and the strength of their research and control organizations, which benefit from the support of international partners (*13*).

Sustaining and consolidating the advances made in controlling the disease, including those made in areas of low endemicity, will depend on retaining political interest and public-health resources. Surveillance and control programmes must be able to adapt to new epidemiological scenarios, rather than continue the same effort or believe that the current success will be permanent (*14*). Surveillance will be important to detect the emergence of disease in regions previously considered to be free of it, such as the Amazon basin, where transmission would involve wildlife rather than domestic vectors and may include local microepidemics of orally transmitted disease (*15*). Surveillance will be equally important to detect the re-emergence of disease in regions where control had been in progress, in areas such as the Chaco region of Argentina and the Plurinational State of Bolivia, but surveillance may become more complicated owing to extensive extra-domestic populations of the main vectors and focalized resistance to pyrethroid insecticides (*16*).

The movement of Chagas disease to areas previously considered non-endemic, resulting from increasing population mobility between Latin America and the rest of the world, represents a serious public-health challenge. The appearance of Chagas disease in places where health professionals have little knowledge or experience of the disease and its control will have to be addressed (*17*). Vectors with the capacity to transmit *T. cruzi* have been identified since the 18th century along maritime travel routes to parts of Africa, the Middle East, South-East Asia and the Western Pacific, thereby increasing the possibility of transmission in previously non-endemic areas. Expertise in Chagas disease must be maintained.

Parasitological treatment is urgently indicated for anyone in the acute phase and for those in whom the infection has been reactivated due to immunosuppression. In the acute cases, medicine is almost 100% effective and the disease can be completely cured. Efficacy decreases as the duration of the infection lengthens. Additionally, during the late chronic phase, severe cardiac or digestive manifestations may occur that require specific treatment. Side-effects are less frequent the younger the age of the patient. Parasitological treatment is also indicated in babies with congenital infection and in patients in the early chronic phase. In adults, especially those with the indeterminate form, parasitological treatment should be offered, but the potential benefits of the treatment and its long duration should be weighed against its frequent side-effects.

The two medicines used for treatment are benznidazole and nifurtimox. The main contraindications to treatment are pregnancy and kidney or liver failure. Nifurtimox is contraindicated in patients with a background of psychiatric or neurological disorders.

There is no vaccine to prevent Chagas disease. Nevertheless, depending on the geographical area, the following prevention and control tools are useful: vector control (the spraying of insecticides), home improvements (such as plastering walls, installing concrete floors and corrugated iron roofs), personal preventive measures (such as using bednets) and good hygiene practices (when preparing, transporting, storing and consuming food). Another preventive measure is to screen blood donors and, before transplantation, to screen organ, tissue and cell donors and recipients.

Key to preventing vertical transmission is the diagnosis of infected pregnant women and the early detection of infection in neonates (secondary prevention). The prevention of laboratory accidents requires the use of standard safety protocols (that is, wearing laboratory coats, gloves, face masks, caps and glasses), especially when dealing with the trypomastigote form of *T. cruzi* (the human infective form). Microepidemics of orally transmitted disease can be prevented by following good manufacturing practices. In areas with malaria transmission, a new Chagas disease surveillance system has been implemented during 2006–2010. Malaria microscopy technicians have been trained to identify *T. cruzi* parasites in malaria films and, consequently, to detect acute Chagas disease in individual cases, possible foodborne outbreaks and active transmission areas for *T. cruzi*.

Assessment

Sustaining the progress made in controlling Chagas disease will depend on political commitment and the retention of public-health resources. Resolution WHA 63.20, adopted by the Sixty-third World Health Assembly in May 2010, urges Member States where the disease is both endemic and non-endemic to control all transmission routes (namely vectors, transfusion, organ transplantation, and vertical and oral routes) and to integrate the care of patients with all clinical forms of the disease into primary health-care services.

WHO has been requested to facilitate networking at the global level and to reinforce regional and national capacities focused on strengthening global epidemiological surveillance of the disease; to prevent all forms of transmission; and to promote early access to diagnosis and treatment. WHO has also been requested to collaborate with Member States and intergovernmental initiatives with the aim of setting objectives and goals for preventing and controlling the disease; to promote research related to prevention, control and care; to advance intersectoral efforts and collaboration; and to support the mobilization of national and international public and private financial and human resources towards the achievement of these goals.

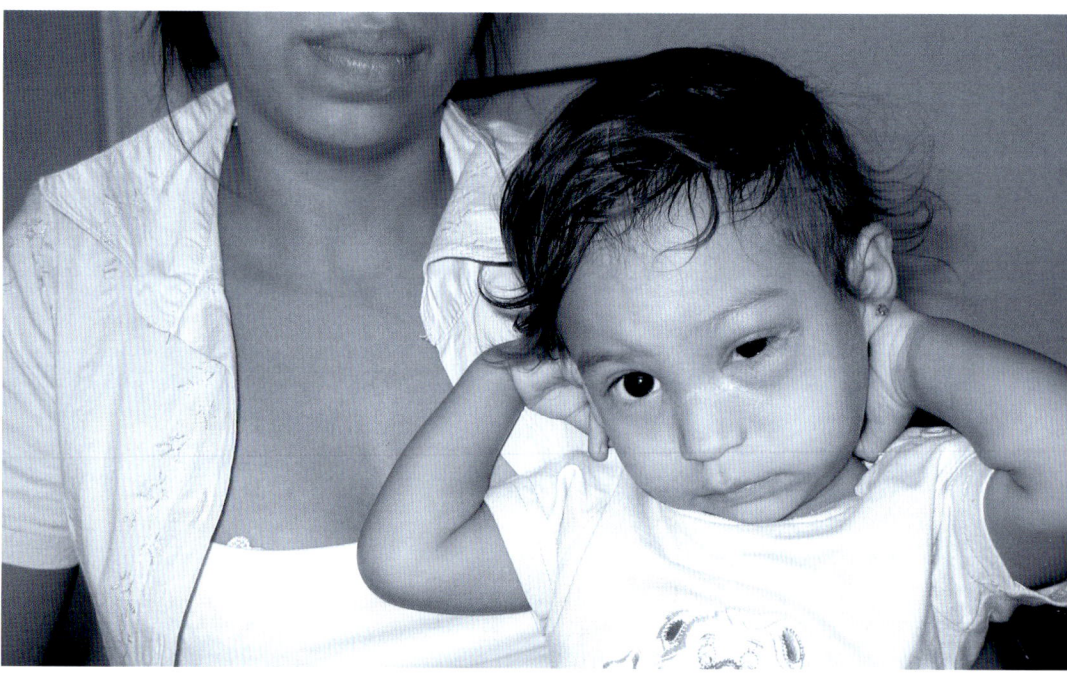

Child presenting Romaña sign waiting to be seen by a doctor in Sonsonate, El Salvador, 2007.

Chagas disease is curable if treatment is initiated soon after infection, but cure rates diminish the longer it takes to tackle the infection. Purplish swelling of both lids of one eye, also called the Romaña sign, is a possible visible mark of acute infection.

© Valladares M - Unidad de vectores SIBASI Sonsonate. Ministerio de Salud Pública y Asistencia Social

REFERENCES

1. Dias E. Estudos sobre o *Schizotrypanum cruzi* [Studies of *Schizotrypanum cruzi*]. *Memórias do Instituto Oswaldo Cruz*, 1934, 28(1):1–110.

2. Wendel S. Transfusion-transmitted Chagas' disease. *Current Opinion in Hematology*, 1998, 5:406–411.

3. Valente SAS, Valente VC, Fraiha Neto H. Considerations on the epidemiology and transmission of Chagas disease in the Brazilian Amazon. *Memórias do Instituto Oswaldo Cruz*, 1999, 94(Suppl. 1):S395–S398.

4. Carlier Y, Torrico F. Congenital infection with *Trypanosoma cruzi*: from mechanisms of transmission to strategies for diagnosis and control. *Revista da Sociedade Brasileira de Medicina Tropical*, 2003, 6:767–771.

5. Chocair PR etal. Kidney transplantation: a new way of transmitting Chagas disease, *Revista do Instituto de Medicina Tropica de São Paulo,* 1981, 23(6):280–282.

6. *Quantitative estimation of Chagas disease in the Americas.* Montevideo, Pan American Health Organization, 2006 (OPS/HDM/CD/425-06).

7. Araujo A et al. Paleoparasitology of Chagas disease – a review. *Memórias do Instituto Oswaldo Cruz*, 2009, 104(Suppl. I):S9–S16.

8. Schmunis GA. Epidemiology of Chagas disease in non endemic countries: the role of international migration. *Memórias do Instituto Oswaldo Cruz*, 2007, 102(Suppl. 1):S75–S85.

9. *Chagas disease control and prevention in Europe. Report of a WHO Informal Consultation (jointly organized by WHO headquarters and the WHO Regional Office for Europe). Geneva, Switzerland, 17–18 December 2009.* Geneva, World Health Organization, 2010 (WHO/HTM/NTD/IDM/2010.1).

10. *Control of Chagas disease: second report of the WHO Expert Committee.* Geneva, World Health Organization, 2002 (WHO Technical Report Series, No. 905).

11. Rassi A, Jr, et al. Development and validation of a risk score for predicting death in Chagas' heart disease. *New England Journal of Medicine*, 2006, 355:799–808.

12. Castillo-Riquelme M et al. The costs of preventing and treating Chagas disease in Colombia. *PLoS Neglected Tropical Diseases*, 2008, 2(11):e336.

13. Dias JC, Silveira AC, Schofield CJ. The impact of Chagas disease in Latin America: a review. *Memórias do Instituto Oswaldo Cruz*, 2002, 97(5):603–612.

14. Schofield CJ, Jannin J, Salvatella R. The future of Chagas disease control. *Trends in Parasitology*, 2006, 22:583–588.

15. Aguilar HM et al. Chagas disease in the Amazon Region. *Memórias do Instituto Oswaldo Cruz*, 2007, 102(Suppl. I):S47–S55.

16. Gürtler RE. Sustainability of vector control strategies in the Gran Chaco Region: current challenges and possible approaches. *Memórias do Instituto Oswaldo Cruz*, 2009, 104(Suppl. I):S52–S59.

17. Jackson Y et al. Management of Chagas disease in Europe. Experiences and challenges in Spain, Switzerland and Italy. *Bulletin de la Société de Pathologie Exotique*, 2009, 102(5):326–329.

5.8 Human African trypanosomiasis (sleeping sickness)

Abstract

Human African trypanosomiasis, or sleeping sickness, is one of the most complex endemic tropical diseases. Spread by the bite of the tsetse fly, the disease flourishes in impoverished, rural parts of Africa. Sleeping sickness is one of the few diseases where effective treatment depends on active screening for the early detection of cases. Symptoms in the initial phase of the illness, when treatment has the greatest chance of success, are often mild or nonspecific. However, patients frequently present for treatment when the disease is already far advanced, when more complex treatment is needed and when its chances of success are jeopardized. Untreated, sleeping sickness is fatal. Death follows prolonged agony.

Description

Human African trypanosomiasis is caused by infection with protozoan parasites belonging to the genus *Trypanosoma*. It is a vector-borne disease and is usually fatal if left untreated. Parasites are transmitted through the bites of tsetse flies (*Glossina* spp.) that have acquired their infection from humans or animals. Following the bite of the infected fly, the parasite multiplies in the lymph and blood, causing headaches, fever, weakness and pain in the joints. Over time, the parasite crosses the blood–brain barrier, migrates to the central nervous system and causes severe neurological and psychiatric disorders leading to death.

The human disease takes two forms, depending on the subspecies of trypanosome involved. *Trypanosoma brucei gambiense* causes a chronic infection that may persist for months or even years without major signs or symptoms of the disease. *Trypanosoma brucei rhodesiense* causes an acute infection; signs and symptoms are observed a few weeks after the infective bite. The acute form develops rapidly, soon invading the central nervous system.

The secure diagnosis of human African trypanosomiasis requires detection of trypanosomes in the patient. Trypanosomes can be present in any body fluid, but they may be difficult to detect owing to the lack of sensitivity of parasitological diagnostic methods and the low number of circulating parasites, especially those belonging to *T. b. gambiense* (*1*). Serological tests are useful only for screening and establishing suspicion of *T. b. gambiense* infection. In some field circumstances, national sleeping sickness control programmes consider a seropositive individual to be infected even in the absence of parasitological confirmation if the suspected case lives in highly endemic or epidemic areas.

Four old, dangerous and cumbersome medicines are registered for the treatment of the disease. Pentamidine is used to treat the first stage of *T. b. gambiense* infection, and suramin is used to treat the first stage of *T. b. rhodesiense* infection. Intravenous melarsoprol is used in the second stage of both forms of the disease; on average, 5% of patients treated with this will have a fatal serious adverse event (*2*). Eflornithine is used in the second stage of *T. b. gambiense* infection. The equipment and solvents required to administer daily treatment with eflornithine for 14 days weigh around 20 kg and cost US$ 618 (US$ 469 for eflornithine and US$ 149 for solvents and equipment). A clinical trial carried out in the Congo and the Democratic Republic of the Congo from 2003 to 2008 has demonstrated that eflornithine can be combined with nifurtimox (registered for Chagas disease) thus reducing the length, the workload and the cost of the regimen (*3*). The combination of eflornithine and nifurtimox has been included in the 16th WHO Model List of Essential Medicines (March 2009). The four registered medicines for treating human African trypanosomiasis plus nifurtimox have been donated to WHO by sanofi-aventis and Bayer Schering Pharma through public–private partnerships. Subsequently, medicines for treatment are distributed free to countries where the disease is endemic by WHO in collaboration with Médecins Sans Frontières Logistique.

Disease distribution and trends

Sleeping sickness is found in remote sub-Saharan areas where health systems are often weak. *T. b. gambiense* is endemic in 24 countries of west and central Africa and causes more than 90% of reported cases of sleeping sickness. *T. b. rhodesiense* is endemic in 13 countries of eastern and southern Africa, representing less than 10% of reported cases. The African Region has the largest proportion of reported cases (90%) and the Eastern Mediterranean Region the remaining 10%. For unexplained reasons, the disease has a focal distribution, and there are areas where tsetse flies are found but sleeping sickness is not. The disease develops in areas ranging from the size of a village to an entire district. Within a given area, the intensity of the disease can vary from one village to the next. Displacement of populations, war and poverty are factors leading to increased transmission.

As with other vector-borne diseases, climate change may affect the extent and distribution of sleeping sickness. Extensive screening in vast areas of historical foci of human African trypanosomiasis in the Sudanese and Guinean ecological zones in west Africa during the past 10 years has not detected cases of the disease. This change appears to have been driven by demographic and climatic dynamics that have reduced the distribution of the tsetse fly in these areas and reduced contacts between people and vectors. Declining rainfall has altered the microhabitats of tsetse flies and also caused decreased cereal production. More land has had to be cultivated for cereals, leading to a loss of tsetse habitat (*4*).

Between 1999 and 2008, the reported number of new cases of the chronic form of human African trypanosomiasis (*T. b. gambiense*) fell by 62%, from 27 862 to 10 372 (*Figure 5.8.1*). Eleven countries (Benin, Burkina Faso, Gambia, Ghana, Guinea-Bissau, Liberia, Mali, Niger, Senegal, Sierra Leone and Togo) reported no cases, and 6 (Cameroon, Côte d'Ivoire, Equatorial Guinea, Gabon, Guinea and Nigeria) reported an average of less than 100 new cases annually. The Central African Republic, Chad, Congo and Uganda each reported 100–1000 new cases annually. Angola, the Democratic Republic of the Congo and Sudan are the most affected countries, with each reporting an average of more than 1000 new cases annually (*5*). During the same period, the number of newly reported cases of the acute form of human African trypanosomiasis (*T. b. rhodesiense*) fell by 58%, from 619 to 259 (*Figure 5.8.2*). Botswana, Burundi, Ethiopia, Namibia and Swaziland reported no cases. Kenya, Mozambique, Rwanda and Zimbabwe reported sporadic cases; Malawi and Zambia reported fewer than 100 new cases each year; Uganda and the United Republic of Tanzania each reported 100–1000 new cases annually (*5*). The number of cases reported annually is considered to be a fraction of the real number of infected individuals. In 2006, the total number of cases was estimated at 50 000–70 000 (*6*).

Fig. 5.8.1 Distribution of human African trypanosomiasis (*T. b. gambiense*), worldwide, 2008

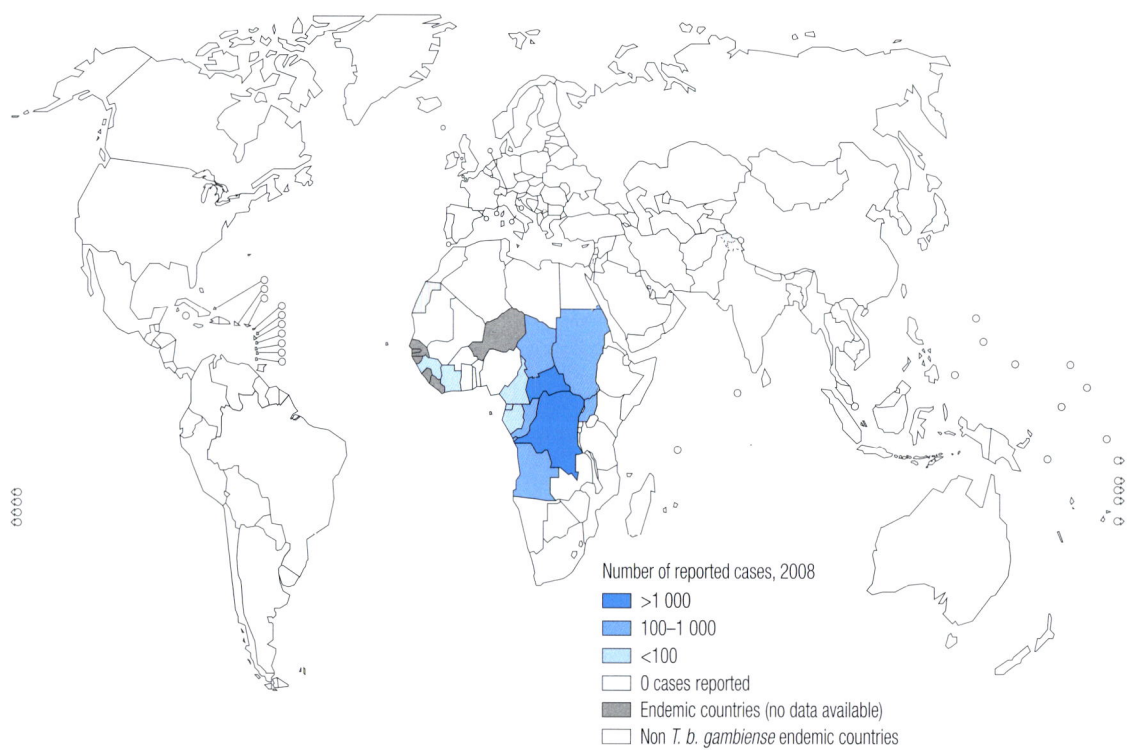

Fig. 5.8.2 Distribution of human African trypanosomiasis (*T. b. rhodesiense*), worldwide, 2008

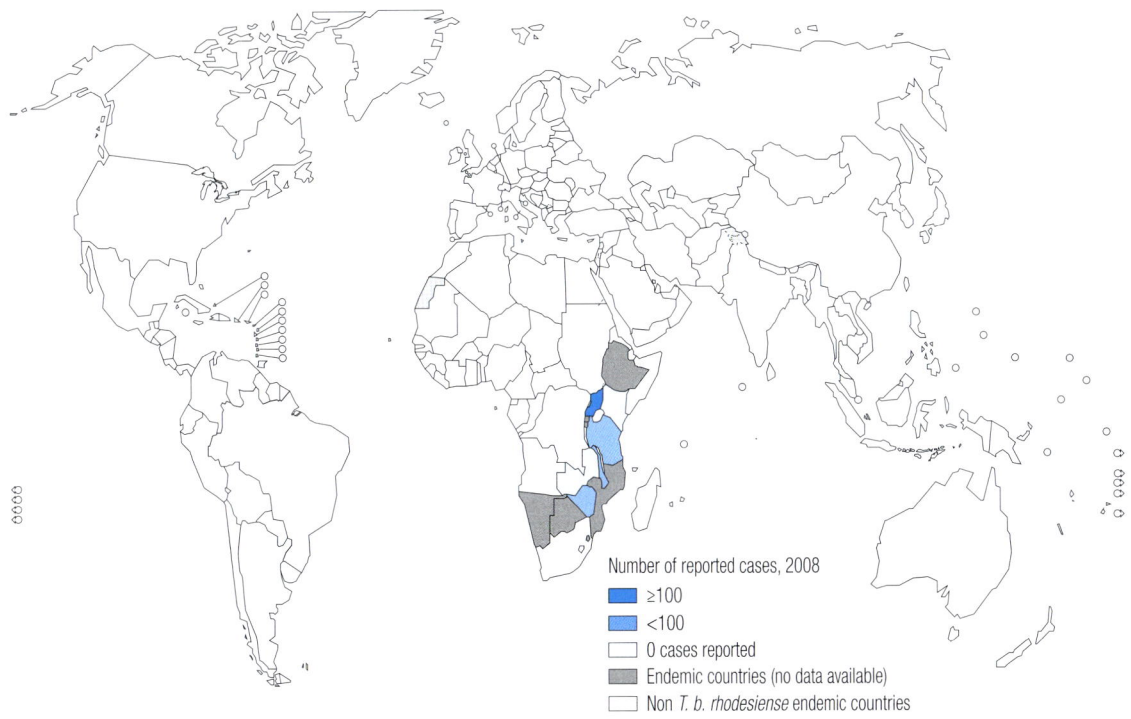

Fig. 5.8.3 Number of new cases of human African trypanosomiasis reported to WHO, worldwide, 1990–2008

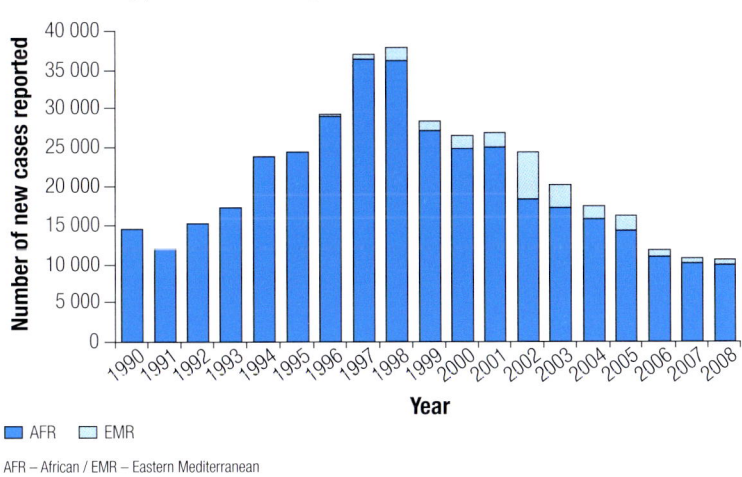

AFR – African / EMR – Eastern Mediterranean

Morbidity

The average course from infection to death is variable but is estimated to last six months for *T. b. rhodesiense* infection and three years for *T. b. gambiense*, unless treatment is provided (*7*). The disease progressively devastates the patient, mainly during the late stage. The patient develops physical and mental disabilities that have a high socioeconomic burden for impoverished families. Stigmatization of patients is common. Neurological and psychiatric sequelae are frequent and permanent. In children, growth and intellectual development are impaired, leading to learning retardation.

Rural populations, living where transmission occurs and depending on agriculture, fishing, animal husbandry or hunting, are most often exposed to the bites of tsetse flies. Although both sexes have the same exposure to risk with regard to farming, women are more likely to become infected during activities related to maintaining the household. Overall, adult men contract more infections because they have more frequent contact with vectors during hunting, fishing and other activities in the forest. The disease can cause amenorrhoea, sterility and abortion, and so contributes to the stigmatization of women. Children are more likely to remain in the village and are less likely to be exposed to infection than adults, but their risk of infection increases when they begin to accompany adults in their activities. Additionally, some childhood activities increase their risk of infection, such as keeping cattle, collecting water, playing in water or travelling to attend a school located outside the village. Congenital transmission of infection is frequent, and the management of infected newborns is complex.

Economic impact

Sleeping sickness, coupled with nagana, the animal form of African trypanosomiasis, has been an obstruction to the development of rural sub-Saharan Africa and a stumbling block to increased production of livestock and agriculture. The FAO estimates that Africa loses US$ 1.5 billion annually in income from agriculture as a result of African trypanosomiasis (*8*). Human disease reduces labour resources, and disease in animals limits the availability of meat and milk and deprives farmers of draught power. The cases of human African trypanosomiasis detected and treated during 1997–2006 averted some 10 million DALYs, mostly due to the prevention of premature death (*8*).

Prevention and control

Even if areas at risk are not completely covered by control and surveillance programmes, most foci of sleeping sickness are well known. Ministries of health carry out interventions, through national sleeping sickness control programmes and health systems. Case-detection and treatment are available in disease-endemic countries, and these benefit from WHO's free supply of reagents, medicines and technical and logistic support. Some foci remain to be fully covered because of security constraints or lack of accessibility.

Given the lack of symptoms during the early stage of the disease, interventions to detect *T. b. gambiense* are based on systematic active screening by mobile teams in endemic areas and supplemented by passive screening at health-care facilities for *T. b. gambiense* and *T. b. rhodesiense* infections. Treatment for early-stage patients could be carried out from the village level to the health–centre level, but the treatment of second-stage disease requires specialized staff in district hospitals. Control activities are complemented in some areas by vector control, mainly implemented within the Pan African Tsetse and Trypanosomiasis Eradication Campaign of the African Union. A memorandum of understanding has been signed between WHO and the Commission of the African Union to coordinate and combine efforts for medical intervention and vector control.

The cost of intervention varies according to the accessibility of the foci but remains high due to the complexity of diagnosing, treating and following up patients. Intervention requires well trained staff and that mobile teams of specially trained health-care workers and specialized treatment services be available. As a consequence of achievements in reducing the number of cases of human African trypanosomiasis in many countries, the priority given to controlling the disease has decreased; this may lead to re-emergence if capacities are not maintained. Resource capacities must be sustained by providing appropriate in-service training. WHO must continue to raise awareness of, and advocate for, keeping control of the disease on the agenda of countries where it is endemic.

Strengthened national health systems will play an increasing role in owning the control of and surveillance for the disease in endemic areas. There is an urgent need to reinforce the capacities of rural health services to allow them to carry out control and surveillance. In addition to the weaknesses of health systems in rural areas where the disease is endemic, the main technical obstacle to control is the lack of appropriate diagnostic tools and medicines. Vector control also needs to be improved and its use encouraged in order to consolidate the achievements of screening and treatment programmes.

Intensification of control activities by national sleeping sickness control programmes under the leadership of WHO and with the support of bilateral cooperation and NGOs has brought about a reduction in the number of cases (*Figure 5.8.3*). Collaboration with partners has improved the accuracy of epidemiological reporting. As a result, WHO is finalizing an atlas of the disease in collaboration with the FAO under the framework of the Programme Against African Trypanosomiasis. The atlas, which includes a village-based distribution of the disease for the past 10 years, will provide a powerful tool to help disease-endemic countries prepare control strategies, carry out interventions and monitor their impact. The atlas will also facilitate evidence-based estimations of at-risk populations and the burden of disease (9).

Since 2007, in an attempt to reduce the treatment fatality rate associated with melarsoprol, efforts have been made to switch to eflornithine by supplying it to national control programmes in a standardized kit along with the appropriate solvents and equipment. The introduction of such a complicated protocol for treatment was supported by ad hoc training provided by WHO. The use of melarsoprol has decreased from 88% of the total second stage cases reported in 2006 to 51% in 2008 (*Figure 5.8.4*) (*10*).

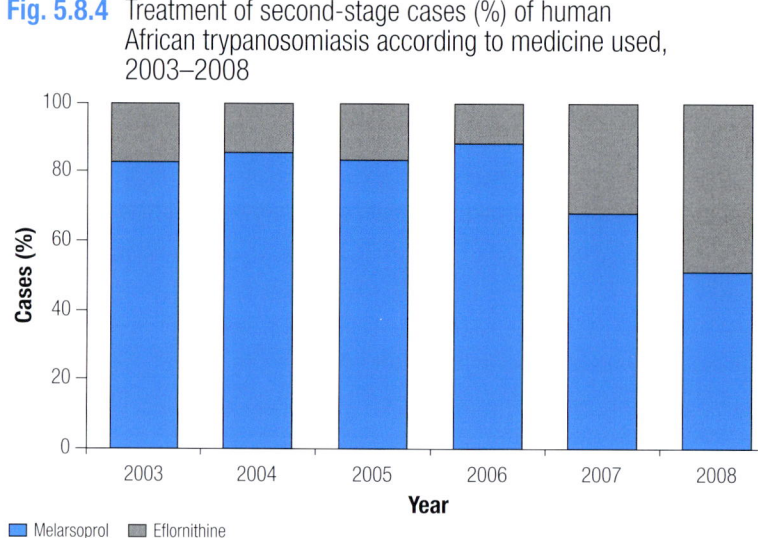

Fig. 5.8.4 Treatment of second-stage cases (%) of human African trypanosomiasis according to medicine used, 2003–2008

The same approach has been introduced for the newly released combination of eflornithine and nifurtimox, again made available with a kit for treatment. These kits are provided by WHO along with systematic in-service training for specialized health-care workers. WHO is playing a major part in developing new medicines by defining the required profile of the medicine, by facilitating clinical trials and by ensuring a distribution system is in place to provide patients with access to new medicines. National control programmes are making efforts to obtain new diagnostics. WHO, in collaboration with partners, has set up a specimen bank for human African trypanosomiasis that is available to research institutions to facilitate the development of appropriate and affordable diagnostic tools.

The main challenge in controlling the acute form of the disease is to control the animal reservoir that represents the risk of permanent transmission and unexpected epidemics. Controlling *T. b. rhodesiense* requires that health systems be strengthened to reduce misdiagnosis and underreporting; there must also be a coordinated multisectoral approach that involves specialists in human and animal health, livestock, agriculture, tourism, wildlife and vector control. Although most of the historical foci of the chronic form of the disease are under control, the challenge will be to sustain the progress made. Improving rural health facilities and ensuring access to new, safe, cheap and easy-to-use diagnostic tools and medicine are crucial to sustaining progress made against this disease.

Assessment

The most immediate challenge is to expand and sustain control and surveillance activities using the best tools available. Research into new tools should be accelerated. Awareness about the disease should be raised, control of the disease should be prioritized and fundraising should be advocated. WHO should continue to support countries and to coordinate the work of all parties concerned with the control of, and research into, human African trypanosomiasis.

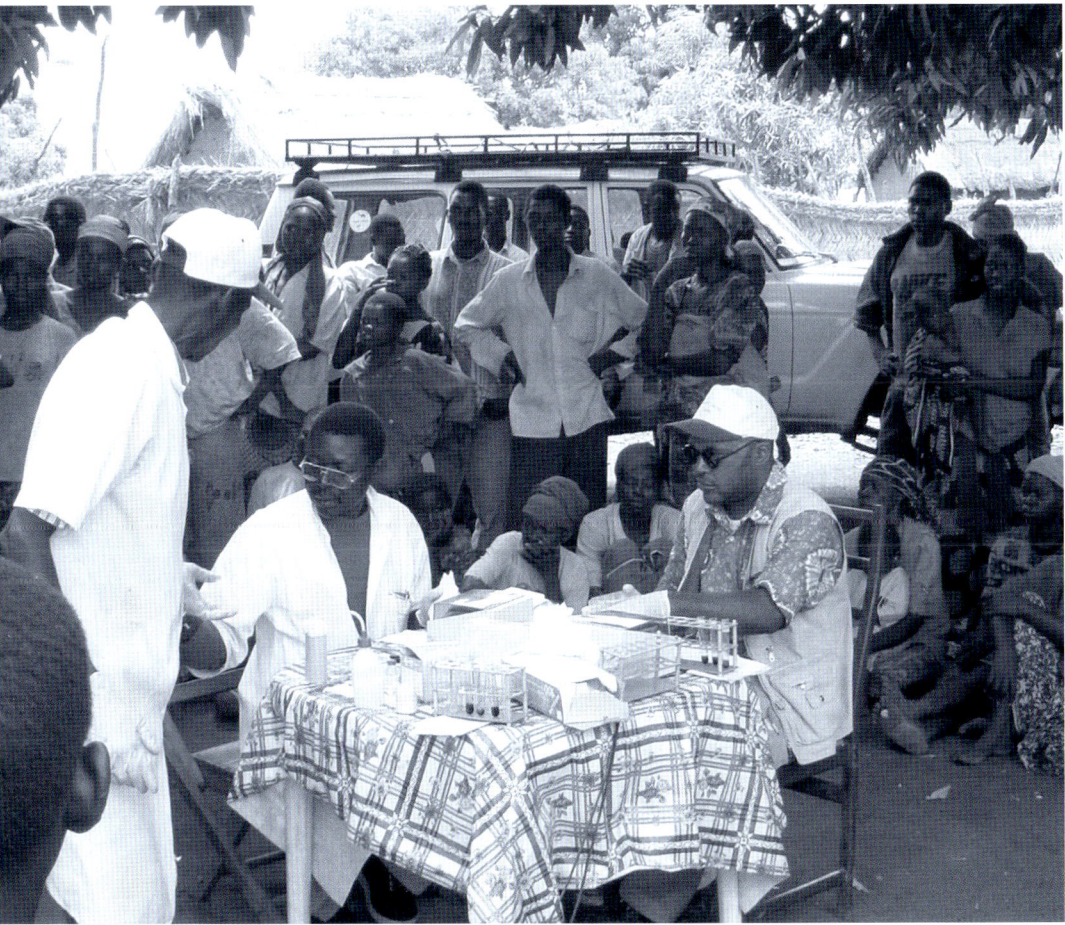

Mobile team of national health care workers performing systematic screening of population for human African trypanosomiasis (sleeping sickness) in Bodo village, Chad.

Confirmation of infection by serological and parasitological tests is always followed by treatment. If untreated the disease is usually fatal.

REFERENCES

1. Chappuis F et al. Options for the field diagnosis of human African trypanosomiasis. *Clinical Microbiology Reviews*, 2005, 18:133–146.
2. *Control and surveillance of African trypanosomiasis: report of a WHO Expert Committee.* Geneva, World Health Organization, 1998 (WHO Technical Report Series, No. 881).
3. Priotto G et al. Nifurtimox-eflornithine combination therapy for second-stage African Trypanosoma brucei gambiense trypanosomiasis: a multicentre, randomised, phase III, non-inferiority trial. *Lancet*, 2009, 374:56–64.
4. Courtin F et al. Sleeping sickness in West Africa (1906–2006): changes in spatial repartition and lessons from the past. *Tropical Medicine and International Health*, 2008, 133:334–344.
5. Simarro PP, Jannin J, Cattand P. Eliminating human African trypanosomiasis: where do we stand and what comes next? *PLoS Medicine*, 2008, 5:174–180.
6. Human African trypanosomiasis (sleeping sickness): epidemiological update. *Weekly Epidemiological Record*, 2006, 81:69–80.
7. Checchi F et al. The natural progression of Gambiense sleeping sickness: what is the evidence? *PLoS Neglected Tropical Diseases*, 2008, 2(12):e303.
8. *On target against poverty: the Programme Against African Trypanosomiasis (PAAT) 1997–2007.* Rome, United Nations Food and Agriculture Organization, 2008.
9. Cecchi G et al. Towards the atlas of human African trypanosomiasis. *International Journal of Health Geographics*, 2009, 8:15.
10. Chappuis F et al. Eflornithine is safer than melarsoprol for the treatment of second-stage Trypanosoma brucei gambiense human African trypanosomiasis. *Clinical Infectious Diseases*, 2005, 41:748–751.

5.9 Leishmaniasis

Abstract

Visceral leishmaniasis predominates in WHO's African, Americas and South-East Asia regions. Cutaneous leishmaniasis predominates in the Eastern Mediterranean and Americas regions; and mucocutaneous leishmaniasis occurs mainly in the Region of the Americas. Cases of visceral leishmaniasis that are not detected or treated cause death within 2 years; untreated cutaneous leishmaniasis may lead to disfiguring scars and stigma. Patients with mucocutaneous disease may also be stigmatized.

Description

Leishmaniasis is a disease caused by protozoan parasites transmitted through the bites of infected sandflies. This disease has a wide range of clinical symptoms. The differing manifestations of the disease arise from infections with different species of *Leishmania*.

Visceral leishmaniasis, also known as kala azar, attacks the internal organs and is the most severe form of the disease. Left untreated, it is usually fatal within 2 years. Furthermore, a percentage of cases may evolve to skin dissemination of parasites. Visceral leishmaniasis is characterized by irregular bouts of fever, substantial weight loss, swelling of the spleen and liver, and pancytopenia. After treatment, this form may evolve into a cutaneous form known as post-kala azar dermal leishmaniasis, which requires lengthy treatment.

The cutaneous form is the most common. It usually causes ulcers on the face, arms and legs. Although the ulcers heal spontaneously, they cause serious disability and leave severe and permanently disfiguring scars. The cutaneous form may produce up to 200 lesions and lead to disability. The patient is left permanently scarred, and so may become socially stigmatized. Diffuse cutaneous leishmaniasis produces chronic skin lesions that never heal spontaneously. Recidivans cutaneous leishmaniasis is a relapsing form that appears after treatment.

The most disfiguring form is the mucocutaneous, which invades the mucous membranes of the upper respiratory tract, causing gross mutilation as it destroys the soft tissues of the nose, mouth and throat. Patients with this form of the disease may also suffer from discrimination and prejudice.

Coinfection with *Leishmania* and HIV is an emerging problem that requires urgent attention. Patients who are coinfected, may relapse repeatedly despite receiving proper treatment, and frequently the outcome is fatal (*1*).

Distribution

Leishmaniasis is a predominantly rural disease, and is prevalent in 88 countries on 4 continents (*Figure 5.9.1, Figure 5.9.2, Figure 5.9.3*). The disease is estimated to cause 1.6 million new cases annually (*2*), of which an estimated 500 000 are visceral (90% of them occurring in Bangladesh, Brazil, Ethiopia, India, Nepal and Sudan) and 1.1 million cutaneous (90% of them occurring in Afghanistan, Algeria, Brazil, the Islamic Republic of Iran, Peru, Saudi Arabia, Sudan and the Syrian Arab Republic) or mucocutaneous (90% occurring in Brazil, Peru and the Plurinational State of Bolivia). Of the 1.6 million estimated cases, only about 600 000 are reported (*2*). Since 1993, the distribution of leishmaniasis has expanded, and there has been a sharp increase in the number of cases recorded (*3*). Since reporting is mandatory in only 33/ 88 affected countries, the true increase in cases remains unknown. The spread of leishmaniasis is mostly caused by voluntary and forced movement of populations that expose non-immune people to infection (*4*). When leishmaniasis occurs in urban areas, conditions often favour explosive epidemics, thereby transforming leishmaniasis from a sporadic threat to an epidemic threat.

Brazil has experienced a sharp increase in the number of cases of visceral leishmaniasis since 1999. Brazil has historically experienced rural epidemics in 10-year cycles, but the disease now appears in urban areas as well. The large-scale migration of people from rural areas to the suburbs of large cities has resulted in densely populated settlements where the newly introduced parasite encounters large numbers of non-immune hosts. Children are the most severely affected. Dogs are the reservoir host for the parasite in Brazil.

In Sudan, in 1997 the number of confirmed cases of visceral disease increased four-fold compared with the previous year. Treatment centres were overwhelmed, and stocks of first-line drugs were depleted. The migration of seasonal workers and the movement of large numbers of people caused by civil unrest carried the epidemic to neighbouring countries.

Although not lethal, epidemics of cutaneous leishmaniasis are of concern in Afghanistan, where war and civil unrest have favoured the spread of the disease and made its control difficult (*5*). The disease flared up in 2002, with 40 000 cases reported in Kabul.

The spread of HIV infection is making people more susceptible to visceral leishmaniasis and changing the epidemiology of the disease. The HIV pandemic in South America, Asia and Africa has expanded into remote areas, and 35/88 disease-endemic countries have already reported cases of coinfection of HIV and visceral disease. In Europe, the number of new cases of visceral disease associated with HIV has declined since the end of the 1990s, mainly as a result of patients having access to antiretroviral therapy. In other parts of the world, where there is insufficient access to antiretroviral therapy, the prevalence of visceral leishmaniasis is rising. In northern Ethiopia, the rate of coinfected patients increased from 19% during 1998–1999 to 34% during 2006–2007 (*1*).

Fig. 5.9.1 Distribution of cutaneous leishmaniasis, worldwide, 2009

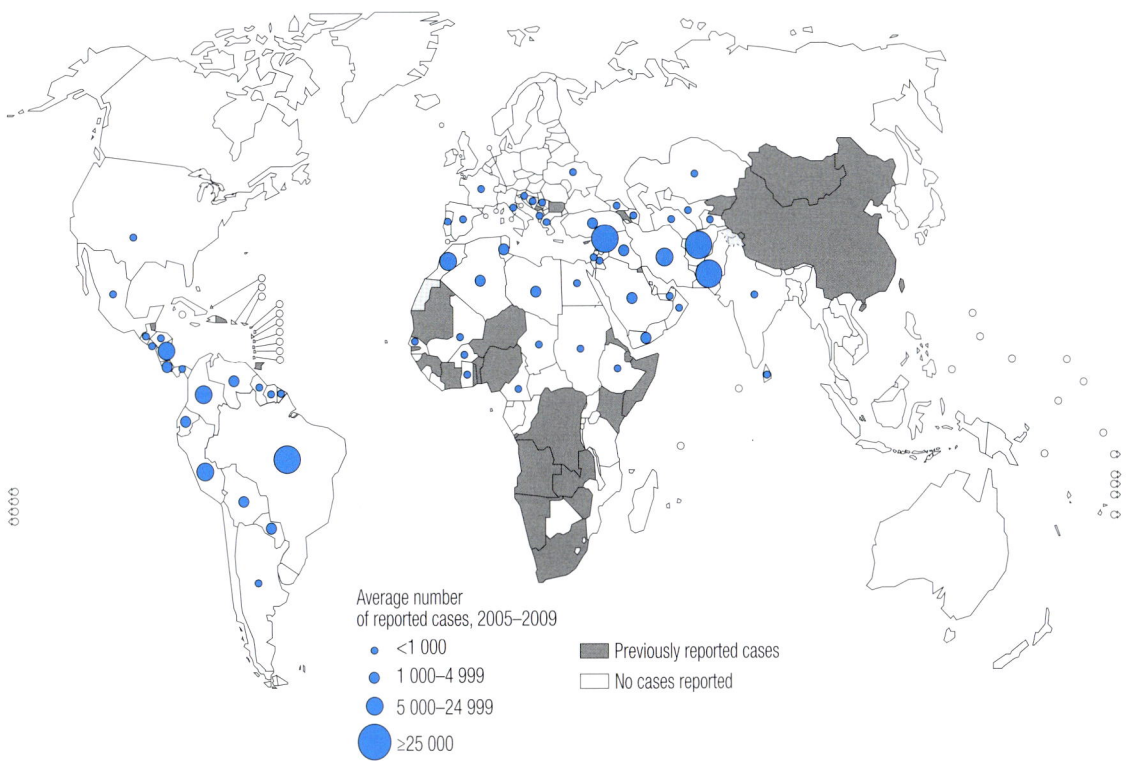

Fig. 5.9.2 Distribution of visceral leishmaniasis, worldwide, 2009

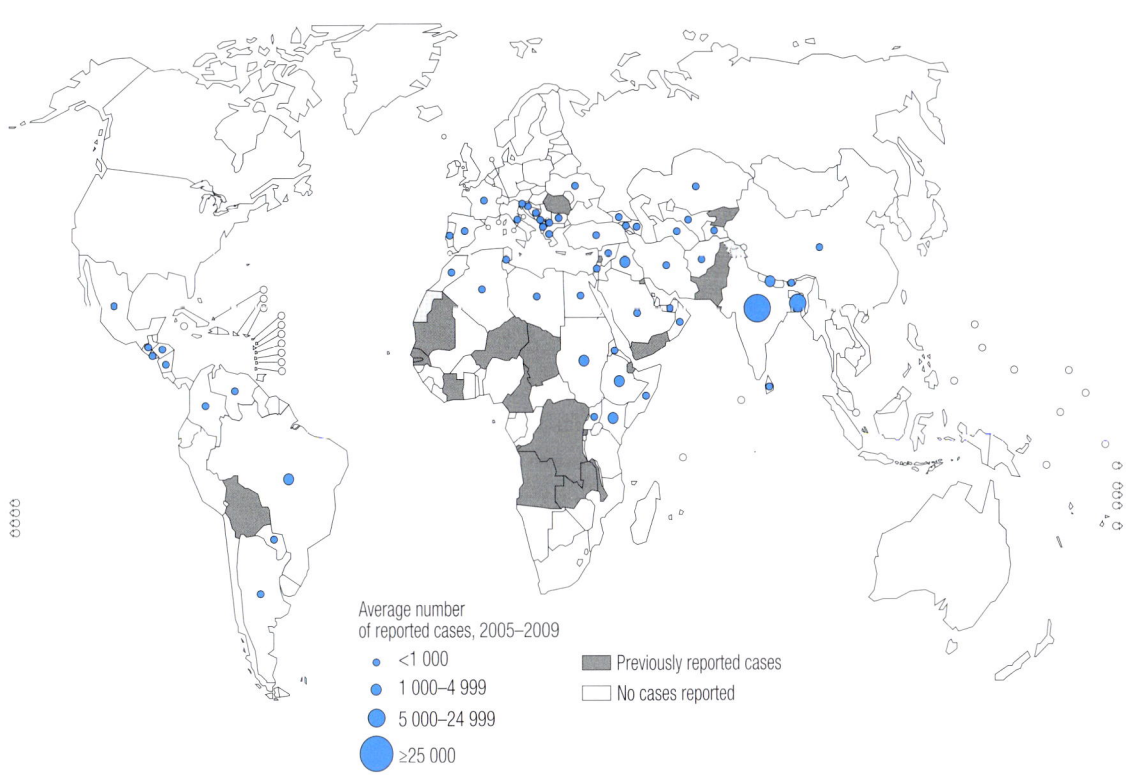

Fig. 5.9.3 Burden of leishmaniasis, by WHO region, 2009

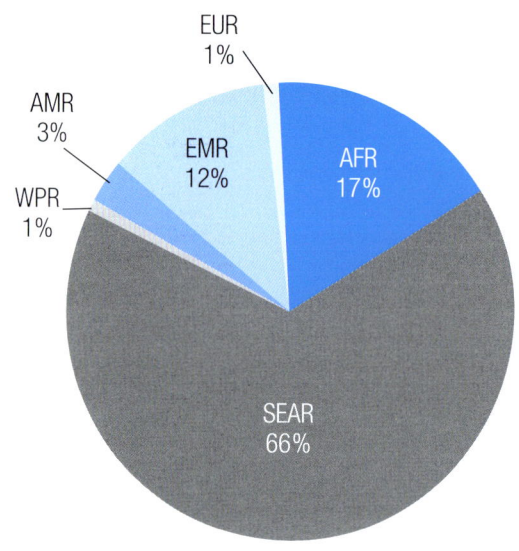

AFR – African / AMR – The Americas / EMR – Eastern Mediterranean / EUR – European / SEAR – South-East Asia / WPR – Western Pacific

Morbidity and mortality

Visceral leishmaniasis may cause large-scale tenacious epidemics with high case-fatality rates (CFRs); about 50 000 people die from the disease annually. In East Africa, particularly in Sudan, epidemics of visceral disease with a high CFR are frequent. Epidemics have occurred recently in Libo Kemkem, Ethiopia (2005); Wajir, Kenya (2007); and in the Upper Nile, southern Sudan (2009), among others.

The true burden of cutaneous leishmaniasis remains largely concealed, partly because those most affected live in remote areas with no access to treatment.

Cutaneous leishmaniasis and mucocutaneous leishmaniasis may lead to patients being excluded from society because many people believe that the disease is contagious. Mothers with cutaneous disease may refrain or be prohibited from touching their children; young women with scars are viewed as being unable to marry (5); and the disease may be the pretext for a husband to abandon a wife.

Decisions about whether to seek care vary depending on the role of the patient within the family (whether the patient is a wage-earner, homemaker, or male or female child), the place of the lesion, the access to care and its affordability, the number of family members suffering from the disease, the perception of treatment's efficacy and, if the patient is a woman, whether she is pregnant.

The sex ratio differs by ecological and cultural setting. Because of occupational exposure to sand flies, there are settings in which men are more affected than women. In other cases, the burden of the disease among women may be underestimated because women have limited access to health facilities.

Prevention and control

For more than 70 years, the first-line treatment in most countries has been injectable pentavalent antimonials. The treatment is lengthy, potentially toxic, and painful; it has become ineffective in parts of India and Nepal as resistance has developed (*6*). In the case of relapse, patients need treatment with a more toxic, second-line medicine, such as amphotericin B or pentamidine. Newly developed, liposomal amphotericin B is highly effective, has almost no side-effects and is now the preferred first-line treatment for visceral disease (*7*). This medicine is too expensive to be widely used by developing countries. Other effective medicines are miltefosine (*8*) and paromomycin (*9*).

Improved control of leishmaniasis will have a major beneficial impact on mortality and morbidity. Where the infection affects only humans, transmission can be reduced by implementing a combination of active case-detection and early treatment. Knowledge of this possibility led to the signing of a memorandum of understanding in 2005 by Bangladesh, India and Nepal to eliminate visceral leishmaniasis by reducing the incidence of the disease to less than 1 case/10 000 individuals by 2015 (*10*).

There is a need to strengthen active case-detection of both cutaneous and visceral disease, and to strengthen the ability to diagnose these at peripheral health centres where patients are usually treated based only on clinical symptoms.

A consensus has emerged that anthroponotic visceral leishmaniasis – which has the potential to develop drug resistance – should be treated with a combination of medicine instead of with monotherapy. Trials of promising combinations of medicine are under way, and it is expected that combination treatment will prevent resistance from developing and shorten the duration of treatment, which, in turn, will make it more likely that patients complete treatment. Combination therapy also will reduce side-effects, be cheaper and allow programmes to be more cost-effective. In 2009, it was recommended that liposomal amphotericin B should be used as an interim strategy until combinations can be implemented. In 2010, this medicine was found to be effective in India in a single-dose regimen; this offers new perspectives for control programmes working in the Indian subcontinent (*11*).

Controlling vectors and reservoirs of hosts are important elements in controlling leishmaniasis. Vector control, using periodic indoor spraying of insecticides, is difficult to sustain; combined campaigns targeting mosquitoes and sand flies are more cost-effective. A suitable alternative to spraying is to use bednets impregnated with long-lasting insecticide. These cost about US$ 5 per unit; and, on average, a treated bednet lasts for 5 years.

Assessment

Bangladesh, India and Nepal, which have the highest burden of visceral leishmaniasis, have decided to reduce the incidence by implementing early case-finding, delivering oral treatment and implementing vector control strategies. In other countries where animal reservoirs sustain transmission there is no cost-effective control strategy. In view of this, WHO has convened an Expert Committee meeting to analyse the situation and recommend appropriate control strategies in line with World Health Assembly resolution WHA60.13 (adopted in 2007).

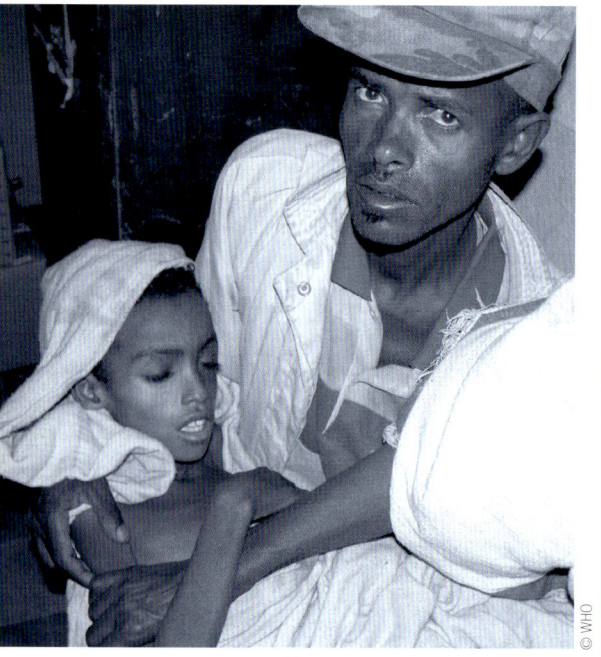

Patient awaiting treatment during a 2005 outbreak in Libo Kemkem, Highlands, Ethiopia.

Visceral leishmaniasis, also known as kala-azar causes irregular bouts of fever, substantial weight loss, swelling of the spleen and liver and anaemia. If untreated, fatality rate can be high.

REFERENCES

1. Alvar J et al. The relationship between leishmaniasis and AIDS: the second 10 years. *Clinical Microbiology Reviews*, 2008, 21:334–359.
2. *The global burden of disease: 2004 update.* Geneva, World Health Organization, 2008.
3. Desjeux P. Worldwide increasing risk factors for leishmaniasis. *Medical Microbiology and Immunology*, 2001, 190(1–2):77–79.
4. Seaman J, Mercer AJ, Sondorp E. The epidemic of visceral leishmaniasis in western Upper Nile, southern Sudan: course and impact from 1984 to 1994. *International Journal of Epidemiology*, 1996, 25:862–871.
5. Reithinger R et al. Anthroponotic cutaneous leishmaniasis, Kabul, Afghanistan. *Emerging Infectious Diseases*, 2003, 9:727–729.
6. Sundar S. Drug resistance in Indian visceral leishmaniasis. *Tropical Medicine and International Health*, 2001, 6:849–854.
7. *Report of a WHO informal consultation on liposomal amphotericin B in the treatment of visceral leishmaniasis.* Geneva, World Health Organization, 2005, (WHO/CDS/NTD/IDM/2007.4).
8. Sundar S et al. Oral miltefosine for Indian visceral leishmaniasis. *New England Journal of Medicine*, 2002, 347:1739–1746.
9. Sundar S et al. Injectable paromomycin for visceral leishmaniasis in India. *New England Journal of Medicine*, 2007, 356:2571–2581.
10. *Regional strategic framework for elimination of kala-azar from the South-East Asia Region (2005–2015).* New Delhi, World Health Organization, Regional Office for South-East Asia (SEA-VBC-85, Rev. 1;a).
11. Sundar S et al. Single-dose liposomal amphotericin B for visceral leishmaniasis in India. *New England Journal of Medicine*, 2010, 362:504–512.

5.10 Cysticercosis

Abstract

Human cysticercosis is caused by the development of *Taenia solium* cysticerci in human tissues. Cysticerci that develop in the central nervous system cause neurocysticercosis. Neurocysticercosis is considered to be a common infection of the human nervous system. Neurocysticercosis is the most frequent preventable cause of epilepsy in the developing world. More than 80% of the world's 50 million people who are affected by epilepsy live in developing countries, many of which are endemic for *T. solium* infections in people and pigs.

Description

Humans acquire cysticerci by ingesting the tapeworm's eggs. Cysticerci also develop in the muscles of pigs that have swallowed *T. solium* eggs. The consumption of undercooked pork by humans completes the tapeworm's life-cycle. The frequency of the disease has decreased in developed countries owing to stricter meat-inspection standards, improved hygiene and better sanitary facilities. Preventing the disease requires strict meat inspection regimens, health education, thorough cooking of pork, sound hygiene, and adequate water and sanitation.

Symptoms include epileptiform attacks, headaches, learning difficulties and convulsions. The location of infection that most often prompts a medical consultation is the central nervous system, followed by the eye and its surrounding tissues. Treating cysticercosis is difficult, and not always successful.

Cysticercosis mainly affects the health and livelihoods of subsistence farmers in developing countries of Africa, Asia and Latin America (*Figure 5.10.1*). Although theoretically amenable to control and declared eradicable by the International Task Force for Disease Eradication in 1993, cysticercosis remains a neglected disease given the lack of information about its burden and transmission, the lack of diagnostic tools available for use in the field, and the lack of validation of simple intervention packages used as part of integrated helminth control strategies.

Fig. 5.10.1 Countries and areas at risk of cysticercosis, 2009

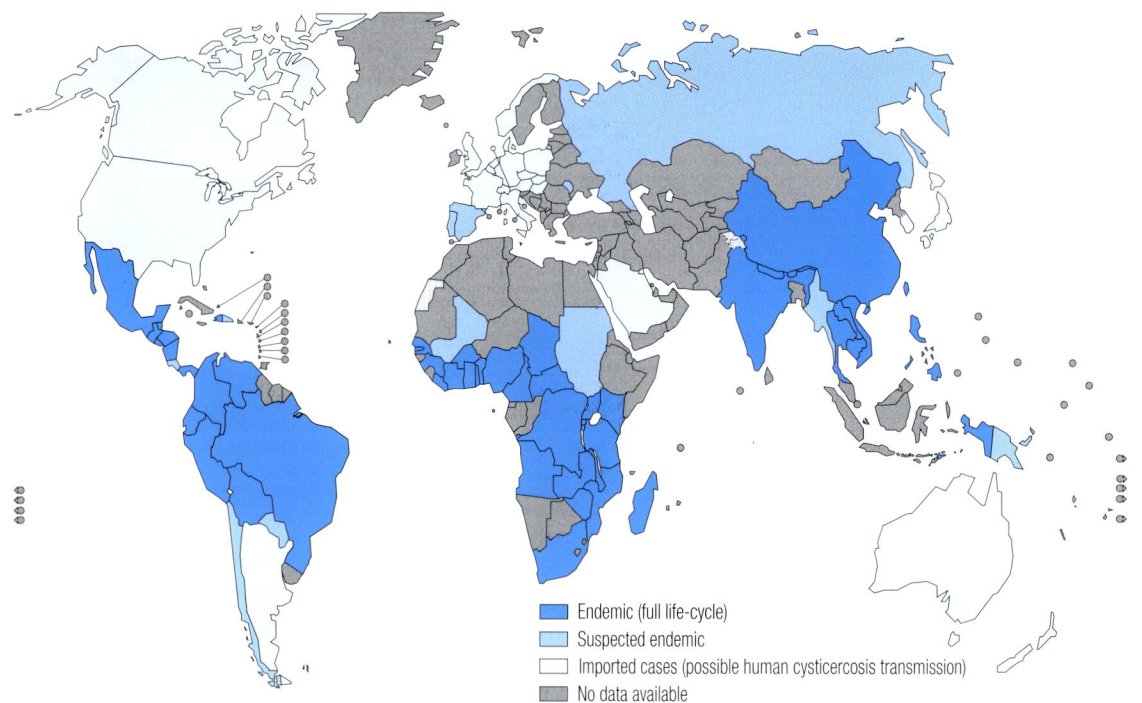

Distribution

Cysticercosis has been a serious problem in Latin America for decades. Hotspots of the disease include the Bolivarian Republic of Venezuela, northern Brazil, Colombia, Ecuador, Guatemala, Honduras, Mexico, Nicaragua, Peru and the Plurinational State of Bolivia. The disease is also endemic in Haiti and possibly the Dominican Republic. Studies in Brazil and the United States indicate that neurocysticercosis is an important cause of human deaths (*1, 2*). In spite of the importance of cysticercosis in WHO's Region of the Americas, surveillance or control programmes have been only rarely established.

Cysticercosis has emerged as a public-health and agricultural problem in most of sub-Saharan Africa, from Cape Verde to Madagascar, because of the increasing popularity of raising pigs and consuming pork. Exceptions in WHO's African Region include the mainly Muslim countries of Algeria, the Comoros, Mauritania and Niger, as well as in countries with low pork consumption, such as Botswana, the Congo, Gabon and Namibia. Community-based surveys of human and porcine cysticercosis have been undertaken in the following countries where the disease is believed to be prevalent, though mainly with focal distribution: Benin, Burkina Faso, Burundi, Cameroon, the Central African Republic, Chad, Côte d'Ivoire, the Democratic Republic of the Congo, Ghana, Kenya, Madagascar, Mozambique, Nigeria, Rwanda, Senegal, South Africa, Togo, Uganda, the United Republic of Tanzania, Zambia and Zimbabwe (*3-6*). Cysticercosis has received little attention from national and regional authorities. The results of recent studies (*7, 8*) have linked the high prevalence of epilepsy with neurocysticercosis.

The disease is endemic in Bhutan, India, parts of Indonesia (Bali and Papua), Nepal and Timor-Leste; the situation is unknown in Bangladesh, the Democratic People's Republic of Korea and Sri Lanka. Case reports suggest that the disease is endemic in Myanmar and Thailand; a recent survey indicated taeniasis *solium* (presence of adult *T. solium* in human intestine) is common in western Thailand. Cysticercosis occurs in all states in India, although the predominantly Muslim states of Jammu and Kashmir and the affluent state of Kerala report few cases. Neurocysticercosis is the cause of epilepsy in up to 50% of Indian patients presenting with partial seizures; ocular cysticercosis is also common. More than half of patients suffering seizures caused by neurocysticercosis are diagnosed with a solitary cysticercus granuloma. Interestingly, a large proportion of Indian patients diagnosed with neurocysticercosis is vegetarian or does not report consuming pork (*9*). Surveys conducted in 2008 in Indonesia suggest that the incidence of cysticercosis has decreased in Bali; Papua is considered to have one of the highest levels of endemicity in Indonesia.

Cysticercosis has been reported in 29 administrative divisions of China, and in 2004 was included for the first time in the national survey of parasitic diseases. Cysticercosis appears to be highly endemic in the south-west provinces of Sichuan, Yunnan and Guizhou. In mainland China, the results of a meta-analysis of data, from the 1930s to the 2000s, showed that human cases of taeniasis and cysticercosis were found in all 31 provinces, municipalities and autonomous regions in mainland China, and there were 5 epidemic zones. The average incidence of *T. solium* infection in China was 0.112% (range, 0.046–15%); the estimated number of taeniasis *solium* patients was 1.26 million; and the estimated number of cysticercosis cases was 3–6 million. The incidence of cysticercosis varied from 0.14% to 3.2% in endemic areas. The majority of cases occurred among people aged 20–50 years, who accounted for 73% of all cases. The ratio of male cases to female cases was 2.4:1. About 200 000 tonnes of infected pork are discarded annually in China, causing a loss of 1 billion renminbi (about US$ 146 million) (*10*).

Community-based surveys of cysticercosis in Viet Nam have detected foci in villages in the northern part of the country where traditional dishes using raw pork are popular. Post-mortem surveys of pigs indicate that the infection is present in the southern part of Viet Nam. There are no published reports from community-based surveys on cysticercosis in Cambodia, the Lao People's Democratic Republic, Malaysia or the Philippines, but case reports suggest that cysticercosis is probably endemic in those countries.

Given the absence of pig-keeping and pork consumption in the Eastern Mediterranean Region, *T. solium* cysticercosis is not considered to be a problem there except in non-Muslim communities in Egypt and southern Sudan. There are reports of human cysticercosis occurring in more affluent countries in the region; these have been linked to transmission through workers from countries where the disease is endemic.

Morbidity

Morbidity mostly occurs when the cysticerci develop in the brain causing neurocysticercosis. The incubation period is variable, and infected people may remain asymptomatic for years. The cysticerci may evade the host's immune system so that viable cysts with little or no inflammatory reaction are usually not associated with symptoms. When cysts are recognized by the host following spontaneous degeneration or after treatment, an inflammatory reaction may occur; this usually results in clinical symptoms, including chronic headaches, blindness, seizures (epilepsy if they are recurrent), hydrocephalus, meningitis, symptoms caused by lesions occupying spaces of the central nervous system, dementia and even death. In severe cases, neurocysticercosis may be fatal and it has been noted as a cause of death among young adult Hispanics and Latinos in the United States. Oedema around calcified cysticercal granulomas also has been found to cause symptoms. The frequency of sequelae following infection with cysticerci remains unknown. The duration of symptoms associated with neurocysticercosis, and the proportion of patients that will fully recover with or without treatment, are ill-defined. Neurocysticercosis is now considered to be a common helminth infection of the human nervous system and the most frequent preventable cause of epilepsy in the developing world. The disease affects from 20% to 50% of late-onset epilepsy cases globally, and is reported to be a common cause of juvenile epilepsy in certain countries, such as India and South Africa. There are about 35 000 cases of epilepsy associated with neurocysticercosis in the Eastern Cape province of South Africa, and more than 400 000 symptomatic cases in Latin America. The occurrence of the disease in developing countries is expected to increase as the demand for pork grows in countries where *T. solium* is endemic. WHO estimates that at least 50 million people suffer from epilepsy, more than 80% of whom live in developing countries. Approximately one third of all cases of epilepsy occur in regions where endemic *T. solium* is associated with neurocysticercosis.

Economic impact

Cysticercosis has a serious impact on the agricultural systems of pig-producing communities. Cysticercosis is responsible for poor pork quality and the labelling of pig carcasses as condemned, thereby reducing farmers' income. An analysis of the burden of cysticercosis in the Eastern Cape province of South Africa indicated that the cost of the disease in that province ranges from US$ 18 million to US$ 34 million annually (*11*). Epilepsy associated with the infection had the largest overall impact: the proportion of patients seeking care and the proportion of time lost from work had substantial influence on the costs. The agricultural costs of cysticercosis in the province were found to be low since most people raised pigs for their own consumption; 76% of people reported seeing cysts in the pork but most did not know what the cysts were.

In west Cameroon, the number of pigs diagnosed with cysticercosis was estimated at 16 000, corresponding to 5.6% of the pig population. The total annual costs associated with cysticercosis were estimated at US$ 13 million, of which 4.7% were due to losses in pig husbandry and 95.3% to direct and indirect losses caused by human cysticercosis. The monetary burden per case of cysticercosis amounted to US$ 252. The average number of DALYS lost was 9/1000 people per year (*12*).

Prevention and control

One of the main obstacles to controlling and eliminating *T. solium* infection is the lack of reliable epidemiological data on infections in people and pigs. Since cysticercosis and *T. solium* do not lead to sudden large-scale international outbreaks of disease, the problem has not seemed to justify international notification. The infection and disease seem to be better suited to national reporting and surveillance as part of a routine system. Appropriate surveillance mechanisms should enable new cases of human or porcine cysticercosis to be reported to national authorities in order to facilitate the identification and treatment of tapeworm carriers and the people who are in close contact with them.

The infection has not been eliminated from any region by a specific programme, and no national surveillance and control programmes are in place except in China. Options available for detecting human cysticercosis include biopsy of subcutaneous cysts (a common manifestation of cysticercosis in Asia), immunodiagnosis (detection of antibodies or parasite antigens in serum samples) and imaging (radiography, computed tomography and magnetic resonance imaging). Methods for detecting cysticercosis in pigs include the rapid, inexpensive method of detecting lingual cysts, but this has low sensitivity, or more sensitive immunodiagnostic tests and postmortem inspection.

In 2009, all aspects of controlling *T. solium* infections and disease were discussed during an expert consultation on foodborne trematodiasis and taeniasis and cysticercosis held in Vientiane, Lao People's Democratic Republic. The meeting issued guidance that focused on using improved preventive chemotherapy in humans and pigs, and the vaccination of pigs. These tools should be ready for use in the field within 2–3 years. The group further acknowledged that community-led total sanitation (that is, the provision of adequate water and sanitation organized by the community itself) is a novel approach to behavioural change and has the potential to be scaled up with minimal investment (*13*).

Assessment

The elimination of cysticercosis requires improvements in chemotherapy for humans and pigs, and the vaccination of pigs. Neurocysticercosis is the most frequent and preventable cause of acquired epilepsy in developing countries.

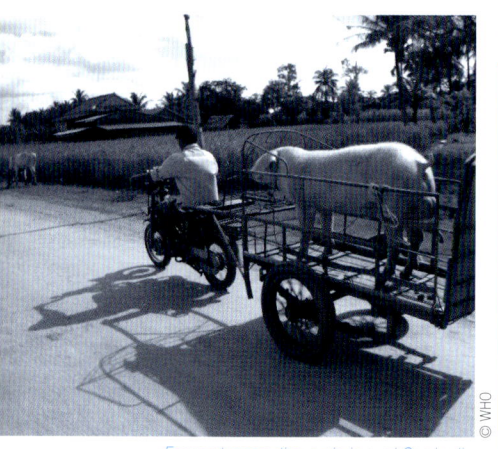

Farmer transporting a pig in rural Cambodia. Cysticercosis has a serious impact on the agricultural systems of pig-producing communities. Cysticercosis is responsible for poor pork quality and the labelling of pig carcasses as condemned, thereby reducing farmers' income.

REFERENCES

1. Flisser A. Epidemiological studies of taeniosis and cysticercosis in Latin America. In: Craig P, Pawlowski Z, eds. *Cestode zoonoses: echinococcosis and cysticercosis. An emergent and global problem*. Amsterdam, IOS Press, 2002:3–11 (NATO Science Series. Series I: Life and Behavioural Sciences, Vol. 341).
2. Sorvillo FJ, DeGiorgio C, Waterman SH. Deaths from cysticercosis, United States. *Emerging Infectious Diseases*, 2007, 13:230–235.
3. Andriantsimahavandy A et al. Situation épidémiologique actuelle de la cysticercose à Madagascar [Epidemiological situation of cysticercosis in Madagascar]. *Archives de l'Institut Pasteur de Madagascar*, 2003, 69(1-2):46–51.
4. Mafojane NA et al. The current status of neurocysticercosis in Eastern and Southern Africa. *Acta Tropica*, 2003, 87:25–33.
5. Geerts S et al. The taeniasis-cysticercosis complex in West and Central Africa. *Southeast Asian Journal of Tropical Medicine and Public Health*, 2004, 35(Suppl.1):S262–S265.
6. Murrell KD. Epidemiology of taeniosis and cysticercosis. In: Murrell KD, ed. *WHO/FAO/OIE guidelines for the surveillance, prevention and control of taeniosis/cysticercosis*. Paris, OIE, WHO, FAO, 2005:27–43.
7. DeGiorgio CM et al. Neurocysticercosis. *Epilepsy Currents*, 2004, 4(3):107–111.
8. Winkler AS et al. Epilepsy and neurocysticercosis in sub-Saharan Africa. *Wiener Klinische Wochenschrift*, 2009, 121(Suppl. 3):S3–S12.
9. Rajshekhar V et al. *Taenia solium* taeniosis/cysticercosis in Asia: epidemiology, impact and issues. *Acta Tropica*, 2003, 87(1):53–60.
10. Chen Y, Xu L, Zhou X. Distribution and disease burden of cysticercosis in China. *Southeast Asian Journal of Tropical Medicine and Public Health*, 2004, 35(Suppl. 1):S231–S239.
11. Carabin H et al. Estimation of the cost of *Taenia solium* cysticercosis in Eastern Cape Province, South Africa. *Tropical Medicine and International Health*, 2006, 11:906–916.
12. Praet N et al. The disease burden of Taenia solium cysticercosis in Cameroon. *PLoS Neglected Tropical Diseases*, 2009, 3(3):e406.
13. *Report of the WHO Expert Consultation on Food-Borne Trematode Infections and Taeniasis/Cysticercosis. Vientiane, Lao People's Democratic Republic, 12–16 October 2009*. Geneva, World Health Organization, 2010.

5.11 Dracunculiasis (guinea-worm disease)

Abstract

Dracunculiasis (guinea-worm disease) has almost been eradicated, but in 2009 Ethiopia, Ghana, Mali and Sudan reported indigenous cases. WHO has now certified 187 countries and territories as free of dracunculiasis or as having interrupted transmission or being an area where transmission never occurred.

Description

Dracunculiasis is an eradicable disease caused by the parasitic worm *Dracunculus medinensis*. This worm is the largest of the parasites that invade human tissues. When a person drinks water containing infected *Cyclops* (the intermediate host of *D. medinensis*) the worm's larvae are released, and they then migrate through the intestinal wall and develop in the tissues. After about one year, the female worm emerges, usually from the patient's feet, and releases thousands of larvae into water, so repeating the life-cycle. No medicines prevent or heal this parasitic disease, which is the only helminthic disease associated exclusively with drinking unsafe water. An effective personal preventive measure is to use gauze to filter suspected contaminated water to eliminate swallowing the *Cyclops* (a small freshwater crustacean about 1–2 mm long).

Distribution

The disease was widespread at the beginning of the 20th century, but during the 1980s transmission was limited to 20 countries of WHO's African, Eastern Mediterranean and South-East Asia regions.

In 1986, 3.5 million new cases were estimated to occur annually (*1*). Based on active village-based searches, 892 055 cases were reported to have occurred in 1989 (*2*). By 2009, as a result of the intensive efforts to eradicate dracunculiasis, the annual incidence was brought down to 3190 cases, a reduction of more than 99% since 1989 (*Figure 5.11.1*). By the end of 2009, only four countries (Ethiopia, Ghana, Mali and Sudan) had indigenous cases; Sudan accounted for 86% of all cases reported in 2009. The number of endemic villages declined from 23 735 in 1991 to 629 in 2009 (*3–7*).

Morbidity

The emergence of the worm is accompanied by painful oedema, intense generalized pruritus, blistering and an ulceration of the area from which the worm emerges. Perforation of the skin is often accompanied by fever, nausea and vomiting. Ulcers caused by the worm's emergence invariably develop secondary bacterial infections that exacerbate the inflammation and pain, resulting in temporary disability lasting from a few weeks to a few months. In severe cases, a person may become permanently disabled.

Both sexes and people of all ages are equally susceptible to infection with *D. medinensis*, but the risk depends upon ingesting drinking-water containing infected *Cyclops*.

In many countries, the incidence of dracunculiasis coincides with the time of peak agricultural activity, resulting in reduced productivity among farmers. The disease is sometimes referred to that of "empty granaries". School attendance is adversely affected in endemic areas due to absenteeism among children suffering from dracunculiasis.

Prevention and control

Dracunculiasis is on the verge of eradication. This achievement will make it the second infectious disease to be eradicated after smallpox. The sustainable benefits of eradicating dracunculiasis include: (i) preventing an estimated 3.5 million cases occurring annually among some of the poorest people in the world in Africa and Asia; (ii) improving health status, agricultural productivity and school attendance in these areas; (iii) strengthening primary health-care systems through the implementation of interventions to eradicate dracunculiasis; and (iv) increasing access to safe drinking-water for underserved populations. Overall, an estimated 29% increase in economic return for the agricultural sector should follow the eradication of dracunculiasis (*8*).

The eradication strategy adopted by all national eradication programmes and recommended by WHO is based on a combination of the following approaches: (i) conducting regular surveillance through community-based surveillance systems; (ii) implementing intensified case-containment measures; (iii) providing access to safe sources of drinking-water through advocacy of organizations concerned with water issues; (iv) providing vector control by treating potential sources of unsafe water with temephos (Abate®) and distributing filters to strain water that may support *Cyclops* species; and (v) providing information, education and communication to bring about behavioural changes.

Once countries have interrupted transmission, a process for certification is followed. WHO has established the International Commission for the Certification of Dracunculiasis Eradication (*9*). The commission has met seven times and, on the basis of its recommendation, WHO has certified 187 countries and territories as dracunculiasis-free, as having interrupted dracunculiasis transmission, or as being an area where transmission never occurred. *Figure. 5.11.2* shows the status of all countries by endemicity and certification status.

The final goal of eradication remains to be achieved. With the high level of commitment evidenced by governments in the remaining countries, Ethiopia, Ghana and Mali are expected to interrupt transmission by 2010. Interrupting transmission in Sudan, which reported 2733 cases in 2009, is likely to take a few years longer. Recurring episodes of insecurity in endemic areas of southern Sudan and Mali are of major concern to national eradication efforts and to the global campaign.

About US$ 72 million was estimated to be needed for eradication work during 2008–2013. The Bill & Melinda Gates Foundation has pledged US$ 40 million towards this financial need as a challenge grant. The United Kingdom's Department for International Development has joined with a pledge of £10 million to cover part of the shortfall. The Carter Center and WHO are campaigning to secure funds to fill the gap.

Assessment

With a high level of government commitment and the efforts of partner agencies, Ethiopia, Ghana and Mali should be able to interrupt transmission by 2010, which is almost in line with World Health Assembly resolution WHA57.9 urging eradication by 2009. Sudan is likely to need a few more years.

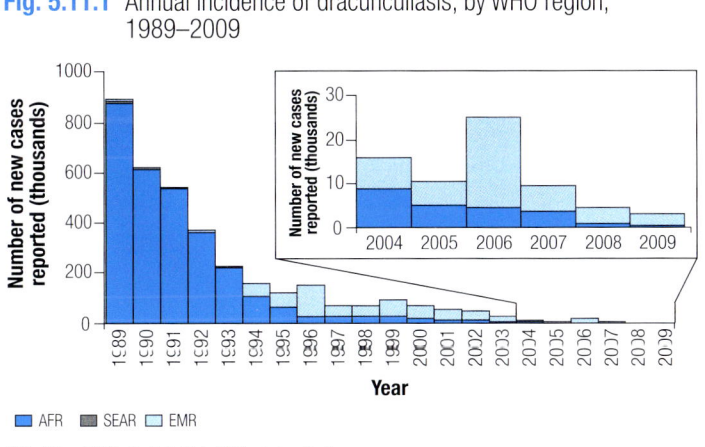

Fig. 5.11.1 Annual incidence of dracunculiasis, by WHO region, 1989–2009

AFR – African / SEAR – South-East Asia / EMR – Eastern Mediterranean

Fig. 5.11.2 Status of dracunculiasis eradication, worldwide, 2010

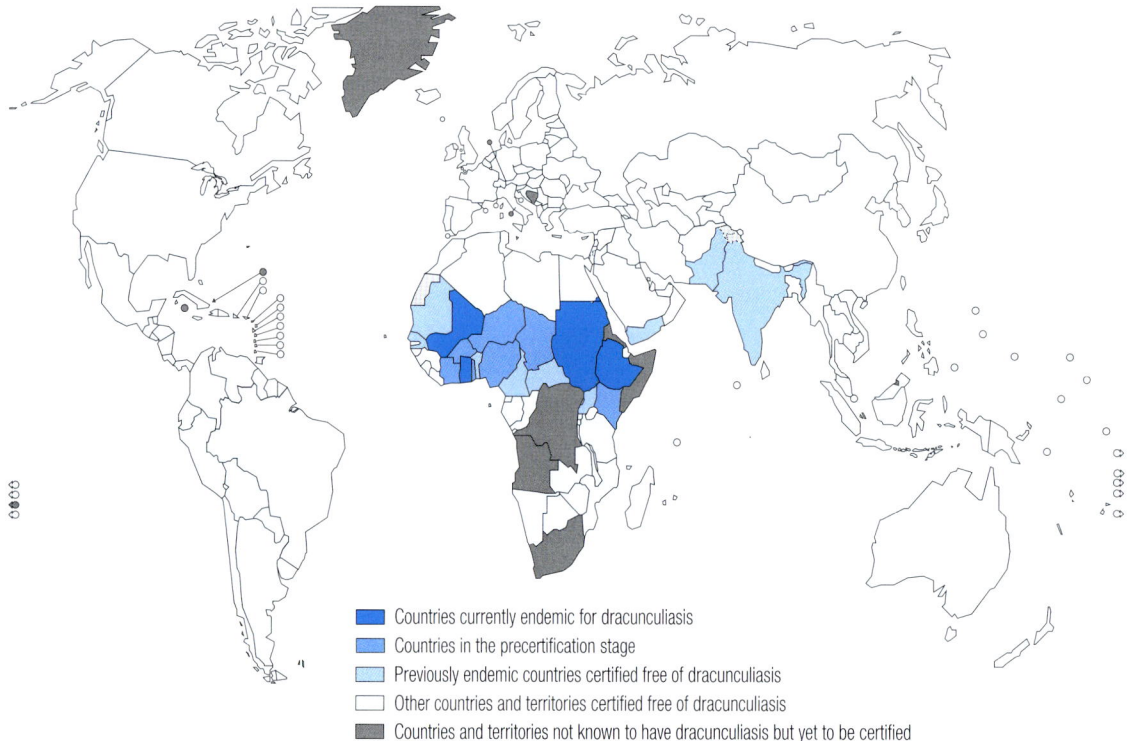

- Countries currently endemic for dracunculiasis
- Countries in the precertification stage
- Previously endemic countries certified free of dracunculiasis
- Other countries and territories certified free of dracunculiasis
- Countries and territories not known to have dracunculiasis but yet to be certified

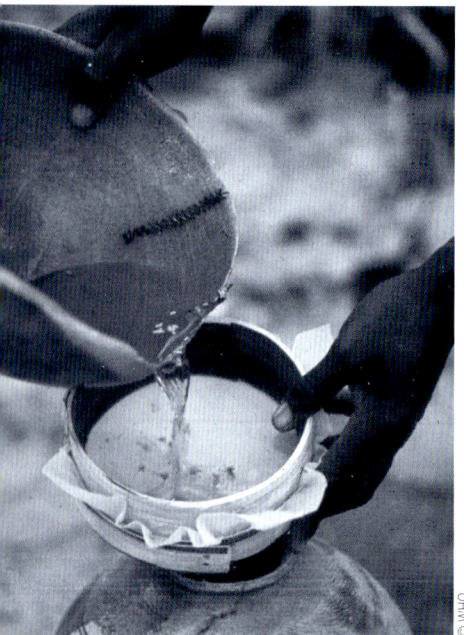

Filtering drinking-water using a fine mesh in Niger. Dracunculiasis (guinea-worm disease) affects people in rural, deprived and isolated communities who have no safe drinking water supply and who depend mainly on open water sources, such as ponds.

REFERENCES

1. Dracunculiasis – global surveillance summary, 1994. *Weekly Epidemiological Record*, 1995, 70:125–132.
2. Dracunculiasis – global surveillance summary, 1992. *Weekly Epidemiological Record*, 1993, 68:125–131.
3. Monthly report on dracunculiasis cases, January–April 2009. *Weekly Epidemiological Record*, 2009, 84:203.
4. Monthly report on dracunculiasis cases, January–May 2009. *Weekly Epidemiological Record*, 2009, 84:280.
5. Monthly report on dracunculiasis cases, January–July 2009. *Weekly Epidemiological Record*, 2009, 84:371.
6. Monthly report on dracunculiasis cases, January–August 2009. *Weekly Epidemiological Record*, 2009, 84:466–467.
7. Dracunculiasis eradication-global surveillance summary, 2009. *Weekly Epidemiological Record*, 2010, 85:165–176.
8. Jim A, Tandon A, Ruiz-Tiben E. *Cost-benefit analysis of the global dracunculiasis eradication campaign*. Washington DC, World Bank, 1997 (Policy Research Working Paper No. 1835).
9. *Certification of dracunculiasis eradication: criteria, strategies, procedures*. Geneva, World Health Organization, 1996.

5.12 Echinococcosis

Abstract

Cystic echinococcosis (hydatid disease) and alveolar echinococcosis develop when humans ingest eggs of *Echinococcus granulosus* or *E. multilocularis*, respectively, which are shed in the faeces of dogs harbouring adult stages of these tapeworms. Echinococcosis has a global distribution, and causes serious morbidity and death if untreated.

Description

Cystic echinococcosis is principally maintained in a dog–sheep–dog cycle. The infection is transmitted to dogs when they are fed infected viscera of sheep or other ruminants during the home-slaughter of animals. Dogs also become infected through scavenging. Direct contact with dogs and consuming vegetables and water contaminated with infected dog faeces are important modes of transmission to humans. Humans are accidental intermediate hosts and are not able to transmit the disease. There are areas of high endemicity in southern South America, the Mediterranean coast, the southern part of the former Soviet Union, the Middle East, south-western Asia, northern Africa, Australia, Kenya, New Zealand and Uganda (*1*).

Human cystic echinococcosis (or hydatidosis) is a disease caused by the larval stages of the dog tapeworm *E. granulosus* (Cestoda). In its domestic transmission cycle, dogs are definitive hosts of the adult tapeworm, and ruminants (particularly sheep and goats) are intermediate hosts. Humans become accidental intermediate hosts following ingestion of eggs through direct contact with definitive hosts or indirectly through food, water or soil contaminated with eggs. The larval stage that emerges from the egg gives rise to a hydatid cyst. A cyst slowly enlarges, and signs and symptoms of disease vary according to its location and size in the body, duration of the development of the cyst, and the cyst type, which is defined according to the classification system of WHO's Informal Working Group on Echinococcosis. Cases of infection with more than one cyst occur. Cysts are found mostly in the liver and lungs, although other organs may be affected. Cystic echinococcosis, a chronic disease with an asymptomatic period of several years, is difficult to diagnose without imaging tools (such as computed tomography or ultrasound); laboratory confirmation of the disease relies on good serological tests. Treatment comprises mainly surgical intervention or percutaneous treatment and/or high dose, long-term therapy with albendazole alone or in combination with praziquantel (*2*). Surveillance in animals is difficult because the infection is asymptomatic in livestock and dogs, and is not recognized or prioritized by communities or local veterinary services.

Distribution

Echinococcosis is widely distributed (*Figure. 5.12.1*). Prevalence and incidence data in animals and humans are variable and, even when the disease is notifiable, its occurrence is frequently underreported (*3*). Given the unreliability of data on human cystic echinococcosis, the figures by country for the collated numbers of cases are estimates based on prevalence of abdominal cysts detected by ultrasound in at-risk rural populations or extrapolated from hospital data mostly collected during special surveys. Data indicate that *Echinococcus* infection is re-emerging as an important public-health issue (*4*).

Human cystic echinococcosis is endemic in parts of east Africa. The disease is present in domestic and wild ungulate populations, and in canids in west and central Africa. The disease is more prevalent in the Nilotic pastoral populations. Between 1981 and 2002, a total of 663 cases (average age 27 years) were operated on in northern Turkana in Kenya (*5*). In that region in 2002, the prevalence in dogs was 33% and in livestock 3–60%. Of 234 cases surgically treated in Addis Ababa, Ethiopia, 94 cases (40%) occurred in Oromiya state. *Echinococcus granulosus* is present in livestock in Somalia but appears not to be a human problem. In 2008, *Echinococcus* isolates from lions in Uganda were shown by DNA analysis to be a separate species (*E. felidis*), the zoonotic potential of which is unknown. Human cases of cystic echinococcosis have occurred in Angola but no data are available.

Echinococcus granulosus is transmitted between dogs and livestock in the major pastoral areas of South America. Human cystic echinococcosis cases occur in Argentina (especially Patagonia), south Brazil (Rio Grande do Sul), Chile, Peru (mainly in the Andes), the Plurinational State of Bolivia (Andes) and Uruguay. The sheep–dog strain (G1 genotype) predominates, while infections with G5, G6 and/or G7 (pig strain) have occurred in Argentina and Chile; infections with G5 (cattle strain) have occurred in south Brazil. Long-term control programmes have been implemented with variable success in south Chile (1979–1997), Uruguay (1965–current) and south-central Argentina (1970–current), although new human cases continue to occur in several regions. In Patagonia, the annual incidence, calculated as the number of surgeries for the disease, was more than 200/100 000 population in Neuquen and Chubut. In Peru, the incidence among humans by administrative department in 2005 ranged from 0 to more than 30/100 000, with a mean of 9/100 000 annually; and the incidence of abdominal ultrasound was 4.7% in highland communities (*6*). Community ultrasound surveys revealed prevalences ranging from 3% to 9% in Andean populations, indicating a significant health burden. Cystic echinococcosis in Brazil is a public-health and economic problem in the southern state of Rio Grande do Sol; the prevalence is 30% in sheep and 11–38% in dogs. *Echinococcus granulosus* occurs rarely in Mexico and Guatemala but is sustained in pig–dog cycles. There are no indications of cystic echinococcosis transmission in Haiti. In central and south America, two other species of tapeworm (*E. vogeli* and *E. oligarthrus*) occur in wildlife cycles and both have zoonotic potential. *Echinococcus vogeli* is more important because domestic dogs become infected by eating rodents (agouti, paca), thereby causing human polycystic echinococcosis (about 150 cases have been described mainly in the Amazonas regions of Brazil and Colombia).

Cystic echinococcosis is endemic throughout WHO's Eastern Mediterranean Region, but data on the disease in humans is fragmented, except in the Islamic Republic of Iran. Cystic echinococcosis is endemic in people and animals throughout the country, while more than 100 cases of human alveolar echinococcosis have occurred in the north-west zone bordering Azerbaijan and Turkey. The prevalence of cystic echinococcosis in humans as detected by ultrasound ranges from less than 0.5% to 1.5%; 1227 cases were surgically treated in three hospitals in Shiraz between 1978 and 1998. Human seropositivity was greater than 5% in the west and south-west of the Islamic Republic of Iran, with 2–18% seroprevalence in nomadic groups (*7*): hydatid control programmes have not been implemented in the country. Cystic echinococcosis is not a major public-health problem in Egypt, but infections in livestock are not uncommon. The incidence of surgery among humans varied from 0.8 to 2.6/100 000, with most cases occurring in Matrouh and Giza governorates. In Sudan, human cystic echinococcosis is mainly a health problem for pastoral tribes in the far south where the ultrasound prevalence in Toposaland during the late 1990s ranged from 0.5% to 3.5%. Human cases have been recorded in Afghanistan, Pakistan and Yemen, but few data have been collected.

Human cystic echinococcosis is endemic throughout southern Europe, Near East, Central Asia and much of central and eastern Russia. Cystic echinococcosis is a public-health problem in Turkey, with an average incidence in humans of 4.7/100 000 annually (range 0.87–20/100 000); 21 303 cases were treated between 1987 and 1994.

Human alveolar echinococcosis is endemic in eastern Turkey (mainly in Kars and Erzurum provinces) with 207 cases recorded up until 1995 (*8*). Human cystic echinococcosis and a few alveolar echinococcosis cases have been reported in Azerbaijan; 484 cases of cystic echinococcosis had been treated surgically over 15 years in Baku up until 2008. Human cystic echinococcosis persists in Albania, the Russian Federation, Tajikistan and Uzbekistan. Alveolar echinococcosis is also present in Kyrgyzstan, the Russian Federation, Siberia, Tajikistan and Uzbekistan.

Cystic echinococcosis is endemic in Bangladesh, Bhutan, India and Nepal, and causes disease in livestock and people. The infection and the disease are assumed to be of low endemicity or absent from Cambodia, Indonesia and the Lao People's Democratic Republic since there is little or no information on echinococcosis in that area. Both cystic echinococcosis and alveolar echinococcosis are endemic in China, with cystic echinococcosis reported in 20/32 provinces or autonomous regions. Eight provinces and autonomous regions of China account for most cases of both cystic echinococcosis and alveolar echinococcosis, with greatest disease burden being in the provinces of Gansu, Qinghai, Shaanxi, Sichuan and in the autonomous regions of Inner Mongolia, Ningxia Hui, Tibet and Xinjiang. Co-endemic transmission occurs particularly in the Tibetan communities of Qinghai and Sichuan. From 2000 to 2002, a survey in Shigu county, Sichuan province, involving 3199 people, found a prevalence of human cystic echinococcosis ranging from 0% to 12% and a prevalence of human alveolar echinococcosis ranging from 0% to 14.3% (9). The incidence of surgery for cystic echinococcosis in parts of Xinjiang and Gansu was 43–80/100 000 population; ultrasound screening surveys revealed prevalence rates ranging between 0.5% to more than 7% in pastoral communities. In Xinjiang, more than 21 000 cases of cystic echinococcosis were treated surgically up until 1995, and estimates for the total number of cystic echinococcosis cases in China run from 347 000 to 1.3 million.

Human alveolar echinococcosis is common in certain rural communities in China, but elsewhere it is generally rare and sporadic. A study published in 2010 suggested that approximately 18 235 new cases of infection (95% confidence interval, 11 900–28 200) occur every year worldwide: 16 629 (91%) in China and 1606 outside China, resulting in a median score of 666 434 DALYs (95% confidence interval, 331 000–1.3 million) (*10*).

Fig. 5.12.1 Distribution of *Echinococcus granulosus* and cystic echinococcosis (hydatidosis), worldwide, 2009

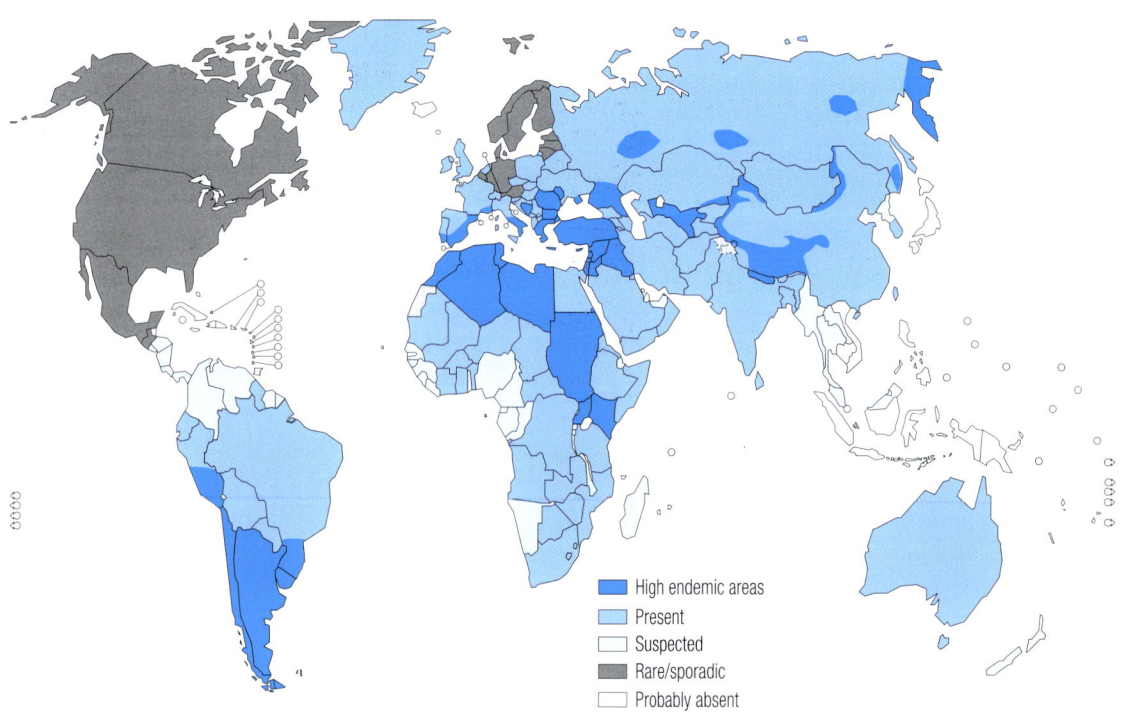

Morbidity

Mortality from cystic echinococcosis ranges between 2% and 4% but it may increase considerably if medical treatment and care are inadequate. Cystic echinococcosis is a health problem for children in endemic regions, and reports of paediatric cases are increasing in some areas. The disease in children is an indicator of the "parasite pressure" in the area, revealing ongoing transmission of infection. In children the disease differs in several aspects from that in adults. Cysts are more frequent in males and the liver and lungs are equally affected. Cysts in children enlarge more rapidly than in adults and cause symptoms earlier, resulting in earlier detection. The so-called rare locations are more commonly detected in children. These include the central nervous system, pelvis, peritoneal cavity, diaphragm, soft tissues, abdominal wall, head and neck region, heart, kidney, spleen, orbit, bone and spine; 50–75% of cases of central nervous system involvement in cystic echinococcosis are reported in children (*11*).

The global burden of cystic echinococcosis has been estimated to be approximately 1 million DALYs (range 860 000–1 175 000), assuming an underreporting of cases. Further estimates indicate that approximately 200 000 new cases are diagnosed annually. The financial burden of the disease in estimates of purchasing power parity is approximately US$ 4.1 billion annually, of which 46% is associated with human treatment and morbidity and 54% with animal-health costs. The burden of human disease of 1 million DALYs is greater than that of several other conditions in the cluster of NTDs, such as dengue, Chagas disease and onchocerciasis, but less than that of trypanosomiasis and schistosomiasis (*12*). Although most cases are associated with direct contact or close association with dogs, an unknown proportion of cases may be associated with contamination of human food and water with canine faecal material.

Prevention and control

Control programmes directed at the regular deworming of dogs combined with public information campaigns and improved post-mortem examinations, the condemning of offal and proper destruction at the slaughterhouse, may eventually be effective. These measures will require at least 5 years and possibly more than 10 years to achieve results, and are expensive and difficult to sustain (*13*). There is no vaccine for dogs, although research is under way (*14*). An effective vaccine for ovine echinococcosis has been developed (*15*) and may become available soon. Community ultrasound surveys have been used to raise awareness in communities considered to be at risk (*16*).

Assessment

Control interventions based on regularly deworming dogs, providing health information and inspecting meat have the potential to reduce the impact of echinococcosis but will take some years to achieve results and will require considerable resources.

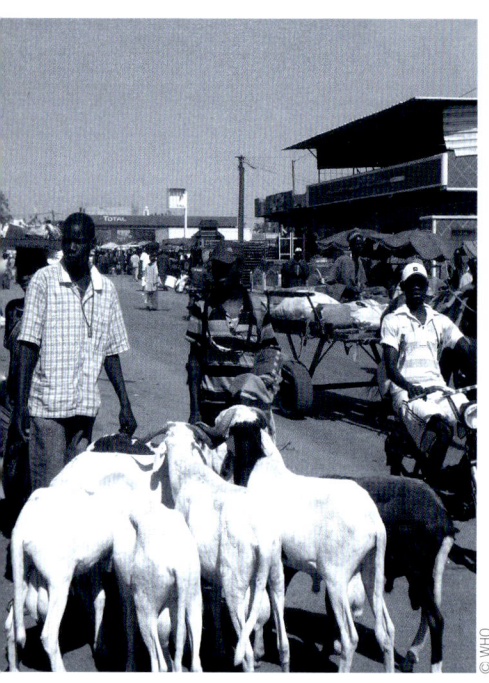

The human-animal interface in a street market scene in Mbour, Senegal.
As many diseases affecting vulnerable populations originate from animals, an integrated human and animal health approach is needed to prevent disease occurrence in humans.

REFERENCES

1. Parasitoses. In: *Hydatidosis in zoonoses and communicable diseases common to man and animals*, 3rd ed. Washington, DC, Pan American Health Organization, 2003, Volume III:184–199.
2. Brunetti E et al. Expert consensus for the diagnosis and treatment of cystic and alveolar echinococcosis in humans. *Acta Tropica*, 2010, 114(1):1–16.
3. Eckert J et al, eds. *WHO/OIE manual on echinococcosis in humans and animals: a public health problem of global concern*. Geneva, World Health Organization and World Organisation for Animal Health, 2001.
4. Jenkins D, Romig T, Thompson R. Emergence/re-emergence of *Echinocccus* spp. A global update. *International Journal for Parasitology*, 2005, 35:1205–1219.
5. Cooney RM, Flanagan KP, Zehyle E. Review of surgical management of cystic hydatid disease in a resource limited setting: Turkana, Kenya. *European Journal of Gastroenterology and Hepatology*, 2004, 16:1233–1336.
6. Gavidia CM et al. Diagnosis of cystic echinococcosis, central Peruvian highlands. *Emerging Infectious Diseases*, 2008, 14:260–266.
7. Sarkari B et al. Human cystic echinococcosis in Yasuj District in Southwest of Iran: an epidemiological study of seroprevalence and surgical cases over a ten-year period. *Zoonoses and Public Health*, 2008, 57(2):146–150.
8. Altintas N. Cystic and alveolar echinococcosis in Turkey. *Annals of Tropical Medicine and Parasitology*, 1998, 92:637–642.
9. Lity et al. Echinococcosis in Tibetan populations, western Sichuan province, China. *Emerging Infectious Diseases*, 2005, 11:1866–1873.
10. Keskin E et al. Hydatid cysts in children [article in French]. *Journal de Chirurgie (Paris)*, 1991, 128(1):42–44.
11. Torgerson PR et al. The global burden of alveolar echinococcosis. *PLoS Neglected Tropical Diseases*, 2010, 4:e722.
12. Budke C, Torgerson P, Deplazes P. Global socioeconomic impact of cystic echinococcosis. *Emerging Infectious Diseases*, 2006, 12(2):296–303.
13. Craig PS, Larrieu E. Control of cystic echinococcosis/hydatidosis: 1863–2002. *Advances in Parasitology*, 2006, 61:443–508.
14. Petavy A et al. An oral recombinant vaccine in dog against *Echinococcus granulosus*, the causative agent of human hydatid disease: a pilot study. *PLoS Neglected Tropical Diseases*, 2008, 2(1):e125.
15. Lightowlers M et al. Vaccination against cysticercosis and hydatid disease. *Parasitology Today*, 2000, 16:191–196.
16. Kachani M et al. Public health education: importance and experience from the field. Educational impact of ultrasound screening surveys. *Acta Tropica*, 2003, 85:263–269.

5.13 Foodborne trematode infections

Abstract

Clonorchiasis, opisthorchiasis, fascioliasis, and paragonimiasis – the commonest forms of foodborne trematode infections – affect millions of people, mainly in Asia. The public-health significance of these infections is gaining recognition; all of them cause significant morbidity, while clonorchiasis and opisthorchiasis lead to cholangiocarcinoma and death if left untreated.

Description

Infections with foodborne trematodes are caused by endoparasitic flukes, which are acquired, generally, through ingestion of food contaminated with the minute larval stages of the worm (metacercariae). Foodborne trematodes are responsible for infections in animals, but many species affect humans as well. The diseases representing the most significant threat to human health are: clonorchiasis (infection with *Clonorchis sinensis*), opisthorchiasis (infection with *Opisthorchis viverrini* or *O. felineus*) and fascioliasis (infection with *Fasciola hepatica* or *F. gigantica*), which all affect the liver and biliary system, and paragonimiasis (infection with *Paragonimus* spp.), which mainly affects the lungs.

Foodborne trematodes have complex life-cycles entailing definitive hosts (humans and animal species that act as reservoirs of infection), a first intermediate host (a freshwater snail) and a second intermediate host (a fish or a crustacean) in which the infective metacercariae develop. *Fasciola* spp. is an exception; its metacercariae are found attached to water plants or float freely in fresh water. All foodborne trematode infections cause diseases that compromise the overall health status of affected individuals and are also responsible for specific and severe organ damage.

Distribution

Fascioliasis is widespread throughout the world, and cases occur on all continents; hot spots are the Caribbean, the Andes, the Mediterranean basin, the Caspian region and south-east Asia. Paragonimiasis has been reported from Africa, south-east Asia and the Americas. Clonorchiasis is limited to eastern Asia; opisthorchiasis is prevalent in eastern and central Asia and in eastern Europe. Within a given country, however, the distribution of foodborne trematode infections is usually focal and limited to specific regions or geographical areas. The focality of transmission mainly reflects behavioural and ecological patterns, such as food habits and the distribution of the intermediate snail hosts.

Foodborne trematode infections have been neglected by the international community. The absence of conclusive information on their geographical distribution and burden means that their public-health impact may have been underestimated for decades. Only a small proportion of those who are infected receive adequate treatment; others are forced to confront chronic disease and, in the most severe cases, death. In 1995, a WHO Study Group estimated that at least 40 million people were infected (*1*). Considering the usual resistance to modifying food habits, which are deeply rooted in the culture and traditions of affected populations, and the fact that these diseases mainly affect marginalized communities not benefiting from social and economic development, it is reasonable to assume that the number of infected individuals is increasing as a consequence of population growth in endemic countries.

Morbidity

Foodborne trematode infections are characterized by a chronic clinical evolution reflecting the steady accumulation of adult worms in the body through subsequent rounds of infection. Early and light infections are usually asymptomatic or only responsible for mild symptoms, such as fever, loss of appetite and fatigue. Fascioliasis is a notable exception and is characterized by a critical acute phase marked by severe abdominal pain, corresponding to the migration of the large parasites through the liver tissues.

As the number of worms increases so does long-standing inflammation of the biological tissues harbouring them. In chronic fascioliasis, inflammation of the larger bile ducts where the adult worms lodge may lead to fibrosis of the surrounding liver tissue and eventually to cirrhosis, ascites and impairment of liver function; anaemia is also a typical finding. In clonorchiasis and opisthorchiasis, the adult worms lodge in the intrahepatic bile ducts; chronic inflammation of the ducts may result in cholangiocarcinoma, a severe malignancy that almost invariably leads to death if not adequately addressed. The clinical picture of paragonimiasis resembles that of pulmonary tuberculosis: chronic inflammation of the lungs associated with severe chest pain, chronic dyspnoea, respiratory failure and expectoration of blood following paroxysmal coughing. Among ectopic cases, cerebral casese are the most severe and may be associated with epilepsy, neurological impairment and dementia.

Differences in age and sex in the epidemiology of foodborne trematode infections are mainly related to food habits. In rural communities in the Republic of Korea, raw fish dishes are typically enjoyed over alcohol: such practices exclude children and are more common among males than females; the epidemiology of clonorchiasis and opisthorchiasis reflects this demographic pattern. In mountainous areas of northern Viet Nam, where catching and eating crabs after summarily roasting them is a common practice among children, severe cases of paragonimiasis may already be encountered in adolescents and young adults. In Egypt, fascioliasis mainly affects girls and young women employed in agricultural work in irrigated plantations where they consume raw vegetables.

Economic aspects

Food safety standards are rarely applied to the small family businesses and informal home fisheries that currently represent an important source of infection for clonorchiasis and opisthorchiasis (2). On the other hand, industrial aquaculture is expanding in developing countries as a way to maintain food security, and the impact on loss of production generated by the associated introduction of food standards is likely to be significant. The case of fascioliasis appears similar since the aquaculture of plants is an increasing source of infection. In addition, given that the main reservoir hosts are livestock (cows, buffaloes, sheep), the impact of fascioliasis on livestock breeding is significant. In the case of paragonimiasis, although most infections occur in remote rural areas and are associated with consumption of wild crabs, the health risk and the consequent economic loss associated with an expansion of aquaculture should not be underestimated.

Prevention and control

Preventive chemotherapy against clonorchiasis and opisthorchiasis has been implemented in the most affected countries, but the scale is limited and not all individuals who need treatment are reached (3). Donated triclabendazole is helping to expand control of human fascioliasis (4). The donation has allowed preventive chemotherapy to be delivered to the most-affected areas and has improved access to individual case-management in less endemic settings. Paragonimiasis remains largely unaddressed, and the scale of treatment activities is limited.

Praziquantel is active against the more common foodborne trematode infections: clonorchiasis, opisthorchiasis and paragonimiasis. Triclabendazole is used to treat fascioliasis and paragonimiasis.

The lack of knowledge about the distribution of these diseases, the underreporting of cases and poor awareness of the public-health significance of foodborne trematode infections have limited the expansion of control activities. In some settings, patients are exclusively dealt with through a case-management approach. No mechanisms for case-detection are in place, and only those individuals who spontaneously present to health centres are treated – that is, those suffering from advanced stages of disease. Access to treatment is limited because medicines are not available or are unaffordable for those infected.

Assessment

Preventive chemotherapy using praziquantel and triclabendazole has been introduced on a limited scale to control the four most common forms of foodborne trematode infections. The use of preventive chemotherapy should be scaled up as should efforts to increase health awareness and improve food hygiene.

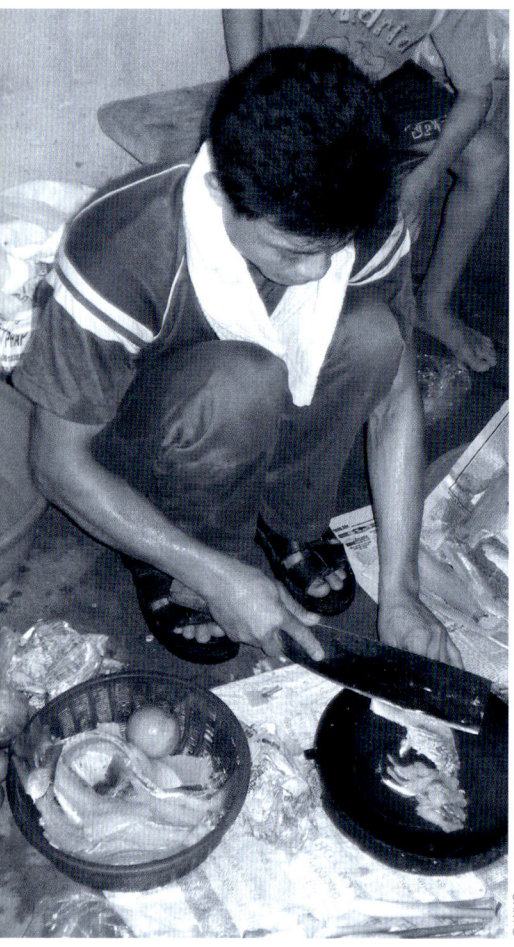

Man cleaning fish in Thanh Hóa province, north central Viet Nam. Consumption of traditional dishes containing raw fresh-water fish is linked with transmission of clonorchiasis and opisthorchiasis.

REFERENCES

1. *Control of foodborne trematode infections. Report of a WHO Study Group.* Geneva, World Health Organization, 1995 (WHO Technical Report Series, No. 849).
2. *Report of the joint WHO/FAO workshop on foodborne trematode infections in Asia. Ha Noi, Viet Nam, 26–28 November 2002.* Manila, World Health Organization Regional Office for the Western Pacific, 2004.
3. *Report of the WHO Expert Consultation on Food-Borne Trematode Infections and Taeniasis/Cysticercosis. Vientiane, Lao People's Democratic Republic, 12–16 October 2009.* Geneva, World Health Organization, 2010.
4. *Report of the WHO Informal Meeting on use of triclabendazole in fascioliasis control. WHO headquarters, Geneva, Switzerland, 17–18 October 2006.* Geneva, World Health Organization, 2007.

5.14 Lymphatic filariasis

Abstract

Lymphatic filariasis arises from infection with mosquito-borne filarial worms. The Global Programme to Eliminate Lymphatic Filariasis, launched by WHO in 2000, has delivered 2.45 billion treatments to people in need to interrupt transmission and control morbidity.

Description

Lymphatic filariasis, which is mostly acquired in childhood, remains silent for a long time after infection. Mosquitoes that bite infected humans transmit the disease. The thread-like, parasitic filarial worms *Wuchereria bancrofti, Brugia malayi* and *Brugia timori* that cause lymphatic filariasis live almost exclusively in humans. These worms lodge in the lymphatic system, the network of nodes and vessels that maintain the delicate fluid balance between the tissues and blood and are an essential component of the body's immune defence system. The worst symptoms of chronic disease generally appear in adults and in men more often than in women: these are damage to the lymphatic system, kidneys, arms, legs or genitals (especially in men) that causes significant pain, large-scale lost productivity and discrimination.

Distribution

Progress has been made in mapping the distribution of lymphatic filariasis during the past decade. Altogether 79/81 endemic countries have initiated mapping the distribution of the disease. Globally, 1334 million people live in the 81 countries where the disease is known to be endemic (*Figure. 5.14.1*). Prior to Global Programme to Eliminate Lymphatic Filariasis, there were an estimated 115 million people infected with *W. bancrofti* and 13 million with *Brugia* spp (*1*). WHO's African and South-East Asia regions harbour 95% of the population living in endemic areas, and 98% of the infected population. Of the endemic population, 874 million (65%) live in the South-East Asia Region (9 endemic countries) and 396 million (30%) live in the African Region (39 countries). The Mekong Plus area (6 countries) accounts for 3%; and the Region of the Americas, Eastern Mediterranean Region and Oceania (with 7, 3 and 17 countries, respectively) together account for 2% (*Figure 5.14.2*) (*2*). All *Brugia* infections are confined to countries of the South-East Asia Region. Ten previously endemic countries have not reported foci and are free from the disease (Burundi, Cape Verde, Rwanda, Mauritius and the Seychelles in the African Region; Costa Rica, Suriname and Trinidad and Tobago in the Region of the Americas; and Brunei Darussalam and the Solomon islands in the Western Pacific Region). Consultations are being held by the international community to develop a mechanism to verify claims that countries are free of the disease.

All countries of the major endemic region – the South-East Asia Region – have initiated mass drug administration, although geographical coverage needs to be extended in Bangladesh, Indonesia, Myanmar, and Timor-Leste. Of the 39 endemic countries in the African Region, 17 have yet to start mass drug administration, and some countries have only limited geographical coverage. The limited progress made in some countries of the South-East Asia and African regions is of immediate concern to the Global Programme to Eliminate Lymphatic Filariasis. At least 10 countries in the African Region are co-endemic for *Loa loa*, and this precludes rapid geographical expansion of the programme because treatment for lymphatic filariasis can cause unacceptable severe adverse events in people infected with *Loa loa*. Modifications need to be made to the use of mass drug administration or other safe treatments for countries where the diseases are co-endemic.

Fig. 5.14.1 Distribution and status of preventive chemotherapy for lymphatic filariasis, worldwide, 2008

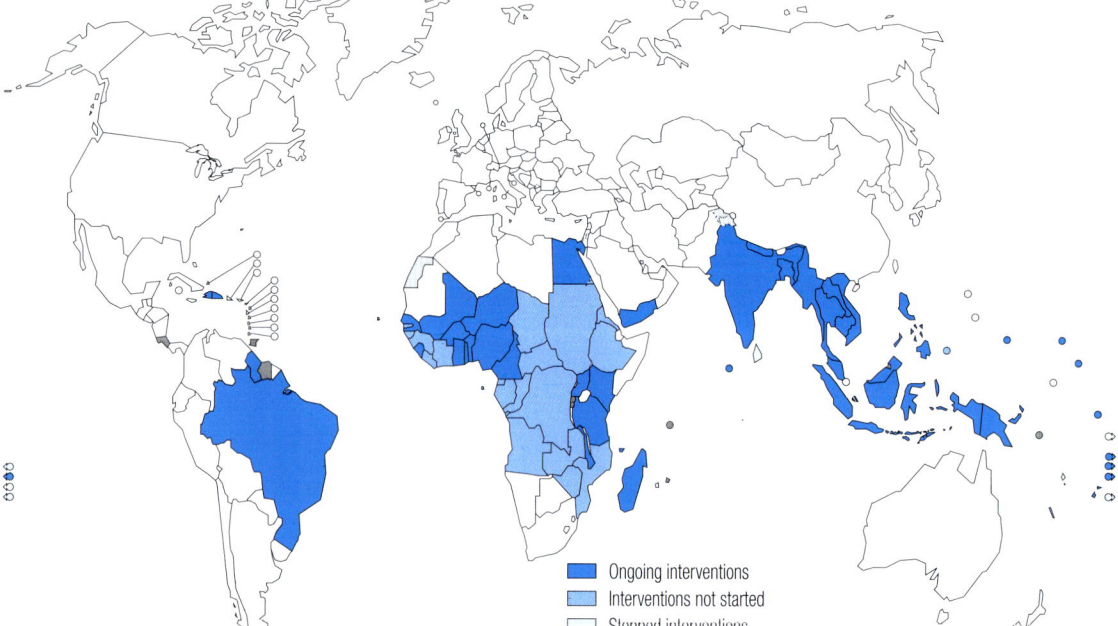

Distribution of lymphatic filariasis is focal in many countries. For the detailed epidemiological situation in countries, please refer to *Preventive chemotherapy and transmission control databank*. Geneva, World Health Organization, 2010 (available at: http://www.who.int/neglected_diseases/ preventive_chemotherapy/databank/en/index.html: accessed January 2009).

Fig. 5.14.2 Distribution of population requiring preventive chemotherapy for lymphatic filariasis, by WHO region, 2008

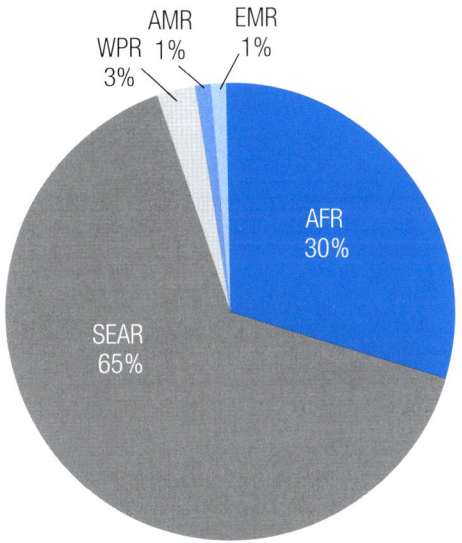

AFR – African / AMR – The Americas / EMR – Eastern Mediterranean / SEAR – South-East Asia / WPR – Western Pacific

Fig. 5.14.3 Reported coverage of treatment (%) for lymphatic filariasis, by WHO region, 2004–2008

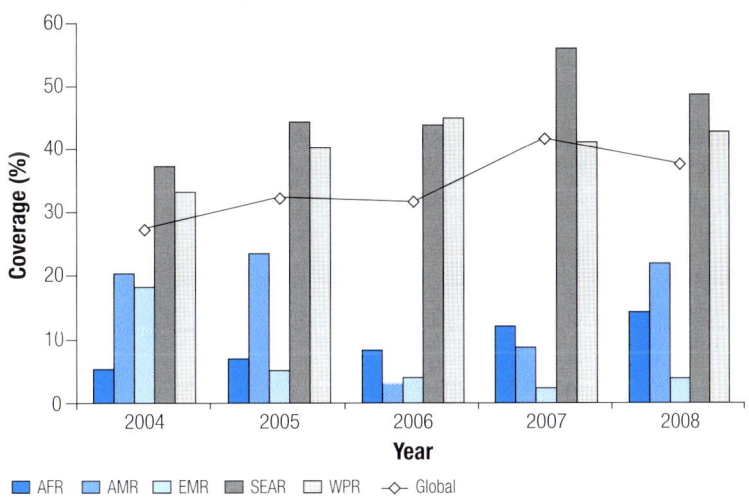

AFR – African / AMR – The Americas / EMR – Eastern Mediterranean / SEAR – South-East Asia / WPR – Western Pacific

Morbidity

Episodes of acute adenolymphangitis and manifestations of chronic disease – especially lymphoedema and elephantiasis of limbs, and hydrocoele – inflict hardship on affected people. Daily chores, occupational activities, educational and employment opportunities, and mobility are severely impaired. The disfigurement of limbs and genital parts leads to stigma, ridicule and psychological distress. Marriage prospects and married life are adversely affected by the disease.

Morbidity management to alleviate disease is a key component of the Global Programme to Eliminate Lymphatic Filariasis. Simple hygiene measures and other measures reduce the frequency of acute episodes and improve lymphoedema. Surgical intervention for hydrocoele is effective and is being offered in more communities. Although 23 countries are implementing case-management programmes, other priorities remain including increasing advocacy, mobilizing resources and orientating health services to make morbidity management and surgical facilities more accessible.

In women the prevalence of lymphoedema and elephantiasis is higher and the impact of disfigurement and disability is more serious. The disease impairs their work and societal roles, which leads to dependence on family and reductions in income and health-seeking opportunities. Women are often discriminated against by the family, community and health facilities, and they experience social isolation and emotional and psychological problems (*3*). Psychosocial counselling and education on coping should be promoted as part of morbidity management programmes.

Prevention and control

The Global Programme to Eliminate Lymphatic Filariasis, which emphasizes the mass distribution of medicines and was launched in 2000 following the adoption of World Health Assembly resolution WHA50.29 in 1997, has enabled many countries to make antifilarial medicines available free to millions of people. Annual mass chemotherapy delivered for 5–6 years is expected to interrupt transmission in many settings and eliminate lymphatic filariasis as a public-health problem. China and the Republic of of Korea made concerted efforts and declared, in May 2007 and March 2008, respectively, to have eliminated the disease as a public-health problem (*4*). At least 9 more countries (the Maldives, Sri Lanka and Thailand in the South-East Asia Region; and the Cook Islands, Kiribati, Malaysia, Niue, Tonga and Vanuatu in the Western Pacific Region) have achieved safe threshold levels of prevalence for microfilaraemia and thus may not require further interventions. Some geographical areas of Burkina Faso, the Comoros, Egypt, Ghana, India, the Philippines and Togo have completed implementation of more than 5 rounds of mass drug administration and achieved significant reductions in the prevalence of microfilaraemia prevalence (*2*). The disease burden is declining in some regions and countries. Improvements in socioeconomic status and the extensive use of personal protection measures against mosquitoes in some countries as well as the use of insecticide-treated bednets for malaria control in parts of Africa are all expected to reduce exposure to transmission and prevalence.

In many settings, children born after the initiation of mass drug administration programmes remain free from microfilaraemia, though a small proportion display circulating antigenaemia and antibodies. Estimates suggest that mass drug administration carried out under the Global Programme to Eliminate Lymphatic Filariasis during 2000–2008 has prevented 8.46 million children aged less than 9 years from acquiring the infection, of which 1.76 million would have developed hydrocoele, 1.06 million would have developed lymphoedema and 5.67 million would have remained subclinical. By 2008, the number of people targeted by mass drug administration programmes had reached 695 million, of whom an estimated 5.63 million thus did not develop hydrocele and 3.38 million did not develop lymphoedema. Preventing disease in all age groups translates to averting 32.46 million DALYs. Mass drug administration offers communities a variety of ancillary benefits. Of the 2.45 billion treatments delivered by the end of 2008, 828 million included albendazole together with diethylcarbamazine or ivermectin thereby preventing and curing other helminthiases, and 63.5 million preschool-aged and school-aged children were treated in 2008 (*3*).

The geographical and population coverage of mass drug administration programmes has been steadily increasing since the Global Programme to Eliminate Lymphatic Filariasis began. By 2009, 53 endemic countries were implementing mass drug administration. The number of people treated has increased from 10 million in 2000 to 546 million in 2007. By the end of 2008, a total of 2.45 billion treatments had been delivered to populations where the disease is endemic (*5*), and this number was approximately 3 billion at the end of 2009. Since 2005, 32–42% of the at-risk population has been treated every year (*Figure 5.14.3*). The proportion and size of the population treated through mass drug administration are likely to be stable at around 35–40% and in the range of 450 million–550 million during the next 3–4 years. The cost of mass drug administration is cheap at US$ 0.05–0.10 per person; the cost of DALY averted per person is US$ 5.90, suggesting that the programme has an advantageous cost–benefit ratio (*6*, *7*).

The timely supply and procurement of medicines of assured quality continues to be an operational priority for the Global Programme to Eliminate Lymphatic Filariasis. The programme will continue its advocacy to strengthen its partnerships, mobilize resources, integrate with programmes to control other NTDs and provide support for research. The next decade of the programme will be crucial and it will need to be initiated in more countries. Mass drug administration will need to be sustained in the countries where it has been implemented; countries on the verge of stopping mass drug administration will need to maintain their surveillance activities.

Assessment

The Global Programme to Eliminate Lymphatic Filariasis, which is based on regularly delivering donated medicines, remains a vital player in efforts to control lymphatic filariasis and interrupt its transmission. Despite significant successes, the date when the goal of eliminating lymphatic filariasis as a public-health problem as set by the World Health Assembly resolution WHA50.29 will be attained cannot be predicted. In many places, lymphatic filariasis persists as a public-health problem.

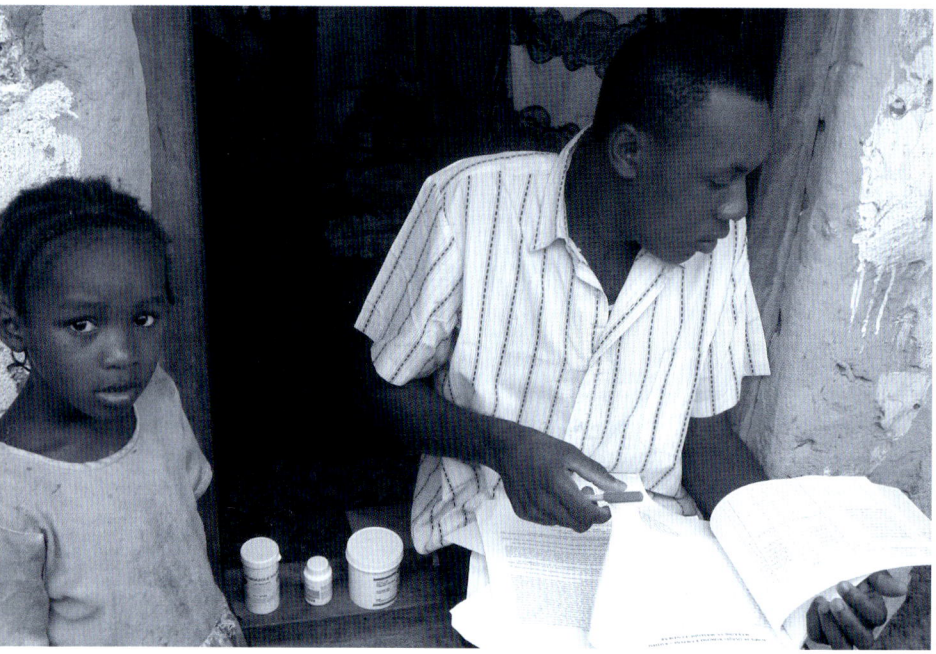

Triple drug administration in Zanzibar: health worker recording treatment with albendazole, ivermectin and praziquantel dispensed to villagers living in areas co-endemic for lymphatic filariasis, schistosomiasis and soil-transmitted helminthiases.

REFERENCES

1. Michael E, Bundy DAP. Global mapping of lymphatic filariasis. *Parasitology Today*, 1997, 13:472–476.
2. Global programme to eliminate lymphatic filariasis: progress report on mass drug administration in 2008. *Weekly Epidemiological Record*, 2009, 84:437–444.
3. *WHO preventive chemotherapy and transmission control databank*. Geneva, World Health Organization, 2010 (http://www.who.int/neglected_diseases/preventive_chemotherapy/databank/en/index.html; accessed July 2010).
4. Global Programme to eliminate lymphatic filariasis: progress report on mass drug administration in 2007. *Weekly Epidemiological Record*, 2008, 37/38:333–348.
5. Person B et al. Health-related stigma among women with lymphatic filariasis from the Dominican Republic and Ghana. *Social Science and Medicine*, 2009, 68:30–38.
6. Ramaiah KD, Das PK. Mass drug administration to eliminate lymphatic filariasis in India. *Trends in Parasitology*, 2004, 20:499–502.
7. Ottesen EA et al. The global programme to eliminate lymphatic filariasis: health impact after 8 years. *PLoS Neglected Tropical Diseases*, 2008, 2(10):e317.

5.15 Onchocerciasis (river blindness)

Abstract

Onchocerciasis is a disease of the skin and eyes caused by a species of filarial nematode (*Onchocerca volvulus*); it is transmitted by blackflies. The disease was brought under control in west Africa through the work of the Onchocerciasis Control Programme (1974–2002). The programme relieved 40 million people from infection, prevented blindness in 600 000 and ensured that 18 million children were born free from the threat of the disease and blindness, thus contributing to the generation of 1 million years of productive labour.

Description

Onchocerciasis, or river blindness, is a parasitic disease caused by a filarial worm (*Onchocerca volvulus*); it is transmitted to humans through the bite of infected blackflies that breed in fast-flowing rivers. The disease causes severe visual impairment, including permanent blindness, and can shorten life expectancy by up to 15 years. Other effects include skin nodules and onchocercal skin disease, which is characterized by skin lesions (severe itching, dermatitis and de-pigmentation). Severe itching alone is estimated to account for 60% of the disease burden.

Onchocerca volvulus is transmitted by vector blackflies of the genus *Simulium*, whose larvae and pupae develop in rapid-flowing, well oxygenated streams and rivers. During blood-feeding, infected blackflies deposit infective larvae, which enter the body; the larvae reach maturity after about a year but may live as long as 14 years. The adult worms in the fibrous nodules of subcutaneous tissue then mate, and females produce microfilariae that migrate to the skin, eyes and other organs. Thousands of microfilariae eventually die in the body, provoking the inflammatory tissue reactions responsible for the disease.

Distribution

More than 99% of people infected with *O. volvulus* live in 30 endemic countries in the African Region; the remainder live in Yemen and 6 countries of the Region of the Americas (the Bolivarian Republic of Venezuela, Brazil, Colombia, Ecuador, Guatemala and Mexico) (*Figure 5.15.1, Figure 5.15.2*). In 1995, 17.7 million people were estimated to be infected, of whom about 270 000 were blind and 500 000 were visually impaired (*1*). Information from rapid epidemiological mapping of onchocerciasis and two cross-sectional studies of the long-term impact of the work of the African Programme for Onchocerciasis Control indicate that these numbers are higher, with nearly 42 million infected people in 1995 and 385 000 who were blind. Furthermore, there were 944 000 cases of low vision and 13.1 million cases of severe itching (*2*).

Prevention and control

The Onchocerciasis Control Programme in west Africa was launched in 1974 with the objective of eliminating onchocerciasis as a disease of public-health importance and an obstacle to socioeconomic development in 7 west African countries. Control was based on aerial application of insecticides to kill the larvae of the vector in riverine breeding sites. Destroying the vector to interrupt transmission needed to continue for about 14 years, since that is the estimated lifespan of the adult worm. Following the donation of ivermectin, mass treatment was included in the Onchocerciasis Control Programme's activities as an adjunct to vector control or as the sole control measure, particularly when the programme was expanded to include 4 additional countries in 1989 (3). The programme was successfully concluded in 2002, although concerns remained about possible recrudescence of onchocerciasis through re-invasion by infected blackflies or migration of infected people in the extended programme area of 11 west African countries; hence the need for the countries to maintain effective surveillance (4).

The African Programme for Onchocerciasis Control was launched in 1995 with the objective of controlling onchocerciasis in the remaining endemic countries in Africa by establishing self-sustaining community-directed treatment with ivermectin. By the end of 2009, 11 600 villages have been surveyed in 19 countries using mapping to determine levels of endemicity. In Mali and Senegal, sustained high coverage of ivermectin alone has eliminated transmission of *O. volvulus* in some foci (5). The African Programme for Onchocerciasis Control is also charged, where possible, with eliminating the vector – and hence the disease – from carefully selected isolated foci using environmentally safe insecticides. *Table 5.15.1* summarizes the achievements of the Onchocerciasis Control Programme in west Africa and the African Programme for Onchocerciasis Control.

The Onchocerciasis Elimination Program for the Americas is a regional initiative that aims to eliminate morbidity related to the disease and interrupt transmission in 6 endemic countries (the Bolivarian Republic of Venezuela, Brazil, Colombia, Ecuador, Guatemala and Mexico), which is distributed in 13 foci. The programme's strategy encourages endemic countries to sustain mass drug treatment with ivermectin every 6 months and aim to reach at least 85% of the 500 000 people at risk of the disease. By the end of 2007, all 6 endemic countries had established effective national programmes in all 13 foci and had treatment coverage of at least 85% twice a year. No new cases of blindness attributable to onchocerciasis have been reported in the Region of the Americas, where eye lesions due to onchocerciasis have been eliminated in 9 of the 13 foci.

Fig. 5.15.1 Distribution of onchocerciasis, worldwide, 2008

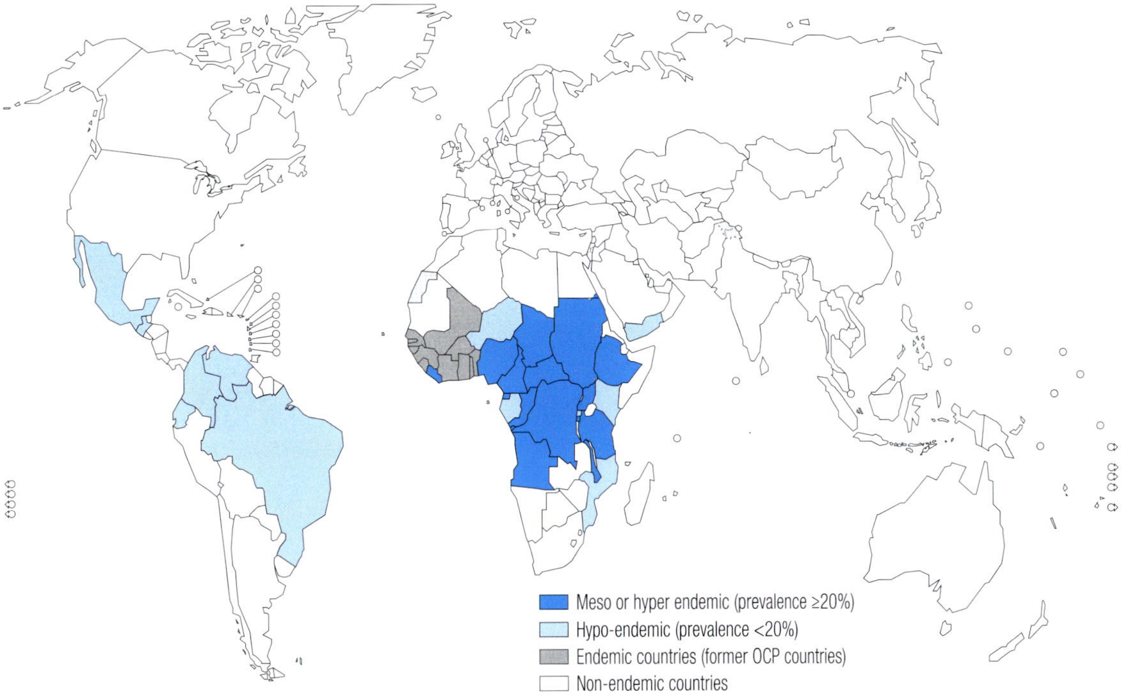

- Meso or hyper endemic (prevalence ≥20%)
- Hypo-endemic (prevalence <20%)
- Endemic countries (former OCP countries)
- Non-endemic countries

Distribution of onchocerciasis is focal in many countries. For the detailed epidemiological situation in countries, please refer to *Preventive chemotherapy and transmission control databank*. Geneva, World Health Organization, 2010 (available at: http://www.who.int/neglected_diseases/ preventive_chemotherapy/databank/en/index.html: accessed January 2009).

Donations of ivermectin have enabled onchocerciasis control to proceed in endemic countries where vector control was impractical, so the African Programme for Onchocerciasis Control was established. Its strategy using community-directed treatment with ivermectin empowers local communities rather than health services to direct the treatment process (*6*). Communities decide whether they want treatment, how to collect and distribute tablets, and how to monitor and record coverage. Health workers provide training and supervision. More than 120 000 communities have responded to this approach and, in 2008, 56.7 million people received ivermectin (*Table 5.15.1*) from nearly half a million community-directed distributors. The cost per treatment is estimated at US$ 0.58 compared with saving US$ 7 per DALY averted. *Table 5.15.2* shows reductions in the prevalence of *O. volvulus* infection and onchocerciasis in areas where in the African Programme for Onchocerciasis Control has used community-directed treatment; the table also shows that the cumulative number of DALYs gained has risen since the project began. A rapid positive impact on human health has been achieved (*2*).

Fig. 5.15.2 Distribution of population requiring preventive chemotherapy for onchocerciasis, by WHO region, 2008

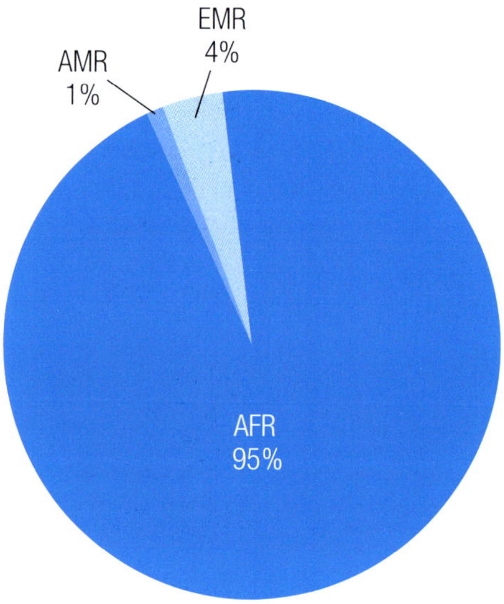

- AFR 95%
- EMR 4%
- AMR 1%

AFR – African / AMR – The Americas / EMR – Eastern Mediterranean

Table 5.15.1 Summary of achievements of the Onchocerciasis Control Programme (OCP) in west Africa and the African Programme for Onchocerciasis Control (APOC), 1974–2008

OCP achievements (1974–2002)	APOC achievements (1996–2008)
40 million people in 11 countries free from infection and eye lesions	20 million cases of severe itching prevented
600 000 cases of blindness prevented	500 000 cases of blindness prevented
18 million children born free of the threat of blindness and debilitating skin disease	120 000 communities mobilized
1 million years of productive labour generated in participating nations	Workforce of 748 000 community-directed distributors of treatment trained and available for other programmes
25 million hectares of abandoned arable land reclaimed for settlement and agricultural production, capable of feeding 17 million people annually	56.7 million people treated in 2008
Economic rate of return of 20%	Economic rate of return of 17% 850 000 DALYs averted per year Cost of US$ 7 per DALY averted

The effort to overcome the public-health significance of onchocerciasis will depend on (i) maintaining high treatment coverage with ivermectin during the lifespan of the adult worm, *Onchocerca,* (ii) supporting government ownership to sustain high treatment coverage (in 2006, governments of 13 APOC countries reported disbursing more than US$ 1 million annually to support core community-directed treatment activities) (7) and (iii) establishing community-directed treatment in post-conflict countries to help strengthen weakened health infrastructure and depleted human resources.

Table 5.15.2 Estimated number of people with *Onchocerca volvulus* infection and clinical manifestations of onchocerciasis in 1995 before the establishment of the African Programme for Onchocerciasis Control (APOC) and during its operations in 2006 and 2008

| Condition or manifestation | Before (1995) | During APOC's operations ||
		2006	2008
Infection	41 894 000	30 724 000	25 719 000
Blindness	385 000	302 000	265 000
Low vision	944 000	809 000	746 000
Severe itching	29 700 000	6 285 000	4 186 000
Cumulative DALYs gained	NA*	3 850 000	5 840 000

*NA, not applicable.

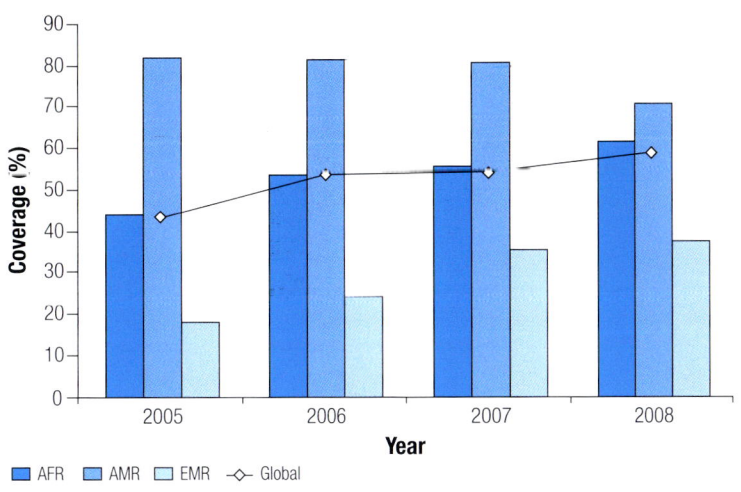

Fig. 5.15.3 Reported coverage of treatment (%) for onchocerciasis, by WHO region, 2005–2008

AFR – African / AMR – The Americas / EMR – Eastern Mediterranean

Assessment

Onchocerciasis control in the African Region is now the responsibility of of the African Programme for Onchocerciasis Control, which was established in 1995. By 2008, 56.7 million people had been treated at a cost of US$ 0.58 per treatment. In the Region of the Americas, the onchocerciasis elimination programme is working to control the infection and development of the disease in the remaining endemic countries.

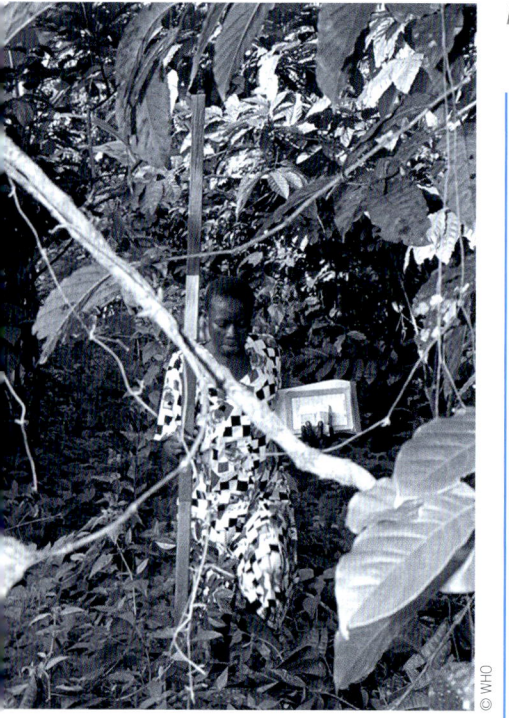

A community drug distributor carrying ivermectin and a dose-pole during an onchocerciasis treatment campaign is making her way to a remote village in Cameroon.

REFERENCES

1. *Onchocerciasis and its control. Report of a WHO Expert Committee on Onchocerciasis Control.* Geneva, World Health Organization, 1995 (WHO Technical Report Series, No. 852).
2. Habbema JDF. *Health impact assessment* [unpublished report]. Erasmus University, Rotterdam and APOC, 2008 (available from the WHO Department of Control of Neglected Tropical Diseases).
3. *Twenty years of onchocerciasis control. Review of the work of the Onchocerciasis Control Programme in West Africa from 1974 to 1994* [internal report]. Geneva, World Health Organization, 1995 (available from the WHO Department of Control of Neglected Tropical Diseases).
4. Sauerbrey M. The Onchocerciasis Elimination Program for the Americas (OEPA). *Annals of Tropical Medicine and Parasitology*, 2008, 102(Suppl. 1):S25–S29.
5. Diawara L et al. Feasibility of onchocerciasis elimination with ivermectin treatment in endemic foci in Africa: first evidence from studies in Mali and Senegal. *PLoS Neglected Tropical Diseases*, 2009, 3(7):e497. doi:10.1371/journal.pntd.0000497.
6. Amazigo UV et al. The challenges of community directed treatment with ivermectin (CDTI) within the African Programme for Onchocerciasis Control (APOC). *Annals of Tropical Medicine and Parasitology*, 2002, 96(Suppl. 1):S41–S58.
7. *Thirteenth Session of the Joint Action Forum, Brussels, Belgium, 4–7 December 2007* [final communiqué]. Ougadoudou, African Programme for Onchocerciasis Control, 2007.

5.16 Schistosomiasis (bilharziasis)

Abstract

Schistosomiasis is now largely confined to sub-Saharan Africa where an estimated 90% of the cases occur. More than 60% of the global burden is confined to 10 countries in WHO's African Region. In the other regions, the disease in humans has been successfully controlled or eliminated.

Description

Schistosomiasis, one form of which is also known as bilharziasis, is a parasitic disease that leads to chronic ill health (*1*). People infected with schistosomes expel the parasite's eggs in their faeces or urine. In villages or communities without proper latrines or sanitation, freshwater resources around the village or community may easily become contaminated with faeces or urine containing the eggs. When they come in contact with water, the eggs hatch and release larvae called miracidia. If the miracidia find the right type of snail, they use it to multiply in several cycles, eventually producing thousands of new parasites, called cercariae, which are then released from the snail into the surrounding water. Humans become infected when they come into contact with skin-penetrating cercariae in water. A child who has suffered persistent and heavy infections is likely to have chronic, irreversible disease later in life, such as liver fibrosis, cancer of the bladder or kidney failure.

Schistosomiasis is characterized as either intestinal or urogenital, depending on where the adult flukes are located. Four species of schistosomes cause the intestinal form (*Schistosoma intercalatum*, *S. japonicum*, *S. mansoni*, *S. mekongi*); in this form the adult worms occupy mesenteric veins, and their eggs pass into the lumen of the intestine and reach the faeces. Adult *S. haematobium,* which cause urogenital schistosomiasis, reside in veins draining the urinary tract, and their eggs normally pass out of the body in the urine. Adult schistosomes are sometimes found in sites other than the intestines or urogenital tract.

Schistosomiasis is diagnosed by identifying specific eggs using parasitological methods, identifying haematuria (for *S. haematobium*), or detecting antibodies or antigens in biological fluids. Imaging techniques are used to detect pathology. Because haematuria is a characteristic of urogenital schistosomiasis, especially in school-aged children, asking people whether they have had blood in their urine can be used to detect communities with a high prevalence of infection.

An estimated 207 million people may have schistosomiasis (*2*). Population growth and the increasing demand for water leads to developments that result in increased transmission and a changing epidemiology of the infection and disease (*3*).

Distribution

Schistosomiasis is endemic in subtropical and tropical areas. Distribution is focal, since transmission depends on specific snail hosts and human activities leading to contamination of water and infection (*Figure 5.16.1*). The snail vectors are of the genera *Biomphalaria* spp. (for *S. mansoni*), *Bulinus* spp. (for *S. haematobium* and *S. intercalatum*), *Neotricula* spp. (for *S. mekongi*) and *Oncomelania* spp. (for *S. japonicum*). Schistosomiasis caused by *S. mansoni* is found in most sub-Saharan countries, in Egypt, the Libyan Arab Jamahiriya and the Arabian peninsular, as well as in Brazil, some Caribbean islands, Suriname and the Bolivarian Republic of Venezuela. *Schistosoma intercalatum* has been identified in the rain forest belt of Africa. *Schistosoma japonicum* is endemic in China, Indonesia and the Philippines. *Schistosoma mekongi* is found in Cambodia and the Lao People's Democratic Republic. *Schistosoma haematobium* is endemic in the Middle East and most of the African continent, including the islands of Madagascar and Mauritius.

Schistosomiasis was endemic in 76 countries (*4*), but transmission has been significantly decreased or interrupted in a number of countries, including the Islamic Republic of Iran, Japan and Tunisia, through the implementation of control interventions. A process for certifying elimination of the disease or interruption of transmission has not yet been put in place.

Schistosomiasis is most prevalent in sub-Saharan Africa, where more than 90% of those who are infected live (*Figure 5.16.2*). About 62% of all cases live in 10 African countries. In the Caribbean islands and Suriname, endemicity has been reduced by development and ecological changes. In the Bolivarian Republic of Venezuela and in Brazil, transmission continues despite achievements made in controlling the disease. In WHO's Eastern Mediterranean Region, control has been successful; and transmission is expected to be interrupted in Egypt, the Libyan Arab Jamahiriya, Morocco, Oman and Saudi Arabia. A control programme has been launched in Yemen; Somalia and Sudan remain the most endemic countries in the region. In the Western Pacific Region, control has been successful in China and it is expected that transmission will be interrupted outside the lake regions (*5*). Schistosomiasis has been controlled in Cambodia (*6*), and interventions are in progress in the Lao People's Democratic Republic. The Philippines has the highest infection rate in Asia but the status of control programmes is unknown.

Neglected tropical diseases in the world today Part 2

Fig. 5.16.1 Distribution of schistosomiasis, worldwide, 2009

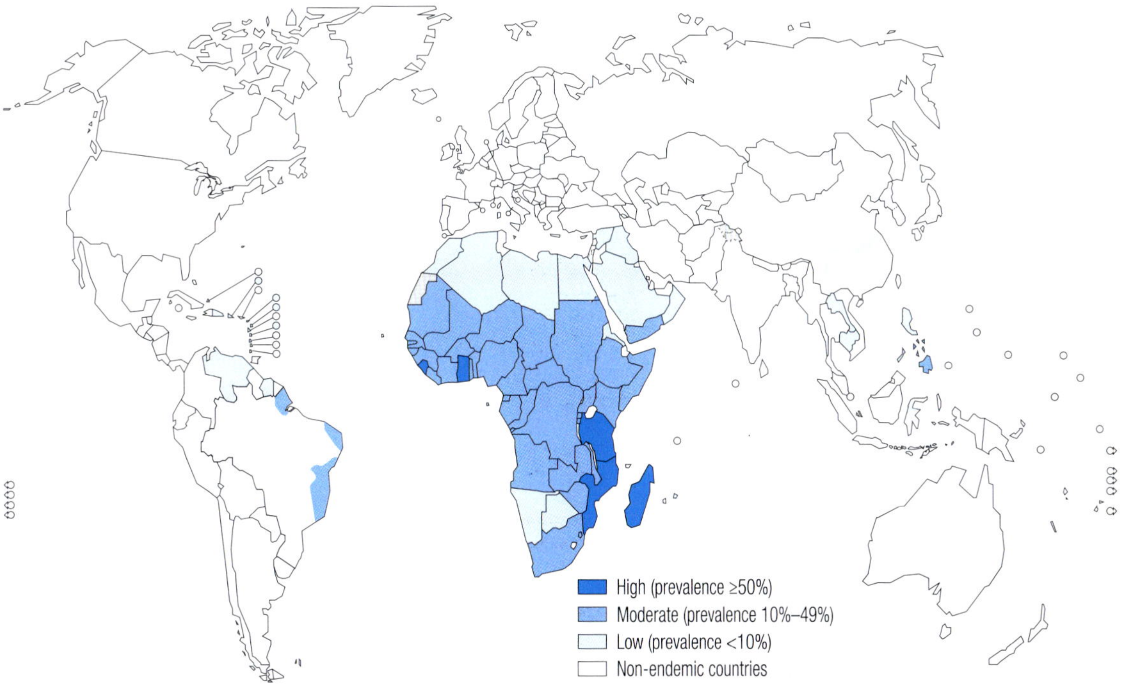

- High (prevalence ≥50%)
- Moderate (prevalence 10%–49%)
- Low (prevalence <10%)
- Non-endemic countries

Distribution of schistosomiasis is focal in many countries. For the detailed epidemiological situation in countries, please refer to *Preventive chemotherapy and transmission control databank*. Geneva, World Health Organization, 2010 (available at: http://www.who.int/neglected_diseases/ preventive_chemotherapy/databank/en/index.html: accessed January 2009).

Fig. 5.16.2 Distribution of population requiring preventive chemotherapy for schistosomiasis, by WHO region, 2008

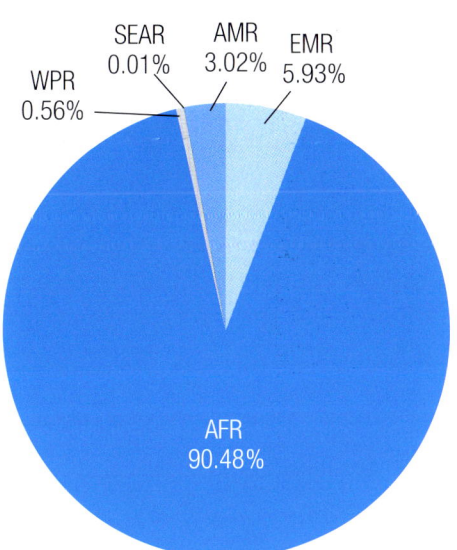

- WPR 0.56%
- SEAR 0.01%
- AMR 3.02%
- EMR 5.93%
- AFR 90.48%

AFR – African / AMR – The Americas / EMR – Eastern Mediterranean / SEAR – South-East Asia / WPR – Western Pacific

131

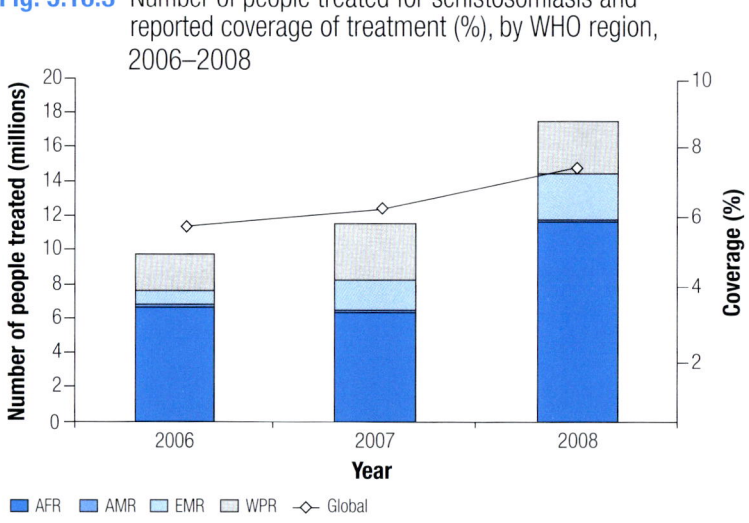

Fig. 5.16.3 Number of people treated for schistosomiasis and reported coverage of treatment (%), by WHO region, 2006–2008

AFR – African / AMR – The Americas / EMR – Eastern Mediterranean / WPR – Western Pacific

Morbidity

The burden of disease caused by schistosomiasis continues to be debated. In 2004, WHO estimated that morbidity caused an equivalent of 1.7 million DALYs (*7*). The disability weight of 0.5% used in WHO's calculations for the average case of infection may be an underestimate; others have estimated greater disability weights (*8*).

Schistosomiasis results in severe organ pathology, anaemia, malnutrition, stunted growth, impaired cognitive development and reduced capacity to work (*9*). Chronic intestinal schistosomiasis progresses from abdominal pain and bloody diarrhoea to hepatosplenomegaly, periportal liver fibrosis and portal hypertension. Urogenital schistosomiasis, which results in haematuria, dysuria, hydronephrosis, calcification of the bladder and other serious sequelae, is also associated with bladder cancer (*10*) and an increased risk of HIV infection (*11*).

The extent of mortality caused by schistosomiasis remains unclear. Using cause-specific reports WHO estimated that 41 000 people die each year (*7*). Analysis of data from sub-Saharan Africa about the relationship between schistosomiasis and specific morbidity were used to estimate that mortality could be as high as 280 000 per year in the African region (*12*). Brazil has demonstrated that implementation of control activities leads to a notable decline in schistosomiasis-related mortality (*13*).

Economic impact

The economic benefits of schistosomiasis control are difficult to quantify, but gains in productivity have resulted from treatment. A study carried out in Cambodia quantified the productivity gained as a result of the national schistosomiasis control programme implemented from 1995 to 2006 (*14*).

The return on investment for each dollar invested was calculated at US$ 3.84. This study also found that the cost per death avoided was US$ 6531, which is comparable to that of other cost-effective interventions, such as distributing insecticide-impregnated bednets and providing childhood vaccination (*14*). In Uganda, the cost effectiveness of the control programme was US$ 3.19 per case of anaemia averted (*15*). Methodological differences in studies on costs and cost effectiveness of control programmes make comparisons difficult. Countries that have been successful in controlling schistosomiasis have also experienced economic development.

Prevention and control

The major intervention used to control the disease is treatment with praziquantel, accompanied by the provision of safe water, adequate sanitation and, where possible, snail control (*1, 2, 5*). Treatment for schistosomiasis has been limited by the availability of praziquantel (*16*). The cost of delivering schistosomiasis treatment has been calculated to be as low as US$ 0.32 in Burkina Faso and as high as US$ 1.02 in Cambodia (*14, 17*). The minimum amount of funds required to provide enough praziquantel to endemic communities in sub-Saharan Africa has been calculated to be US$ 200 million annually (*16*).

Children of school age are the most heavily infected, and treatment targeted at this group prevents future pathology (*18*). Children can be reached through schools, but the proportion of children attending school is often variable, with girls and children from poorer families being underrepresented. Women of childbearing age are excluded from public-health programmes; WHO recommends that women who are pregnant, lactating or of childbearing age should be offered praziquantel during treatment campaigns (*19*).

Donations of praziquantel have enabled treatment to be significantly scaled up in recipient countries. Nevertheless, the major impediment to control is the availability of sufficient praziquantel to achieve full coverage *(16)*. With external help, it will be possible to control schistosomiasis nationally.

Assessment

Reports to WHO *(20)* indicate that of the 17.5 million people treated for schistosomiasis globally in 2008, 11.7 million were in sub-Saharan Africa. Clearly there is an urgent need to provide praziquantel for the other 189.3 million sufferers in Africa. The goal of reaching at least 75% of school-aged children by the end of 2010 as set by resolution WHA54.19, which was adopted by World Health Assembly in 2001, is unattainable (*Figure 5.16.3*). The goal is unattainable because scaling up treatment would mean reaching around 71 million school-aged children, whereas in 2008 only 11.7 million people of all age groups had been reached. The main reason is the limited availability of praziquantel (there was no donated praziquantel until 2008) and the fact that donated praziquantel meets only about 10% of the need.

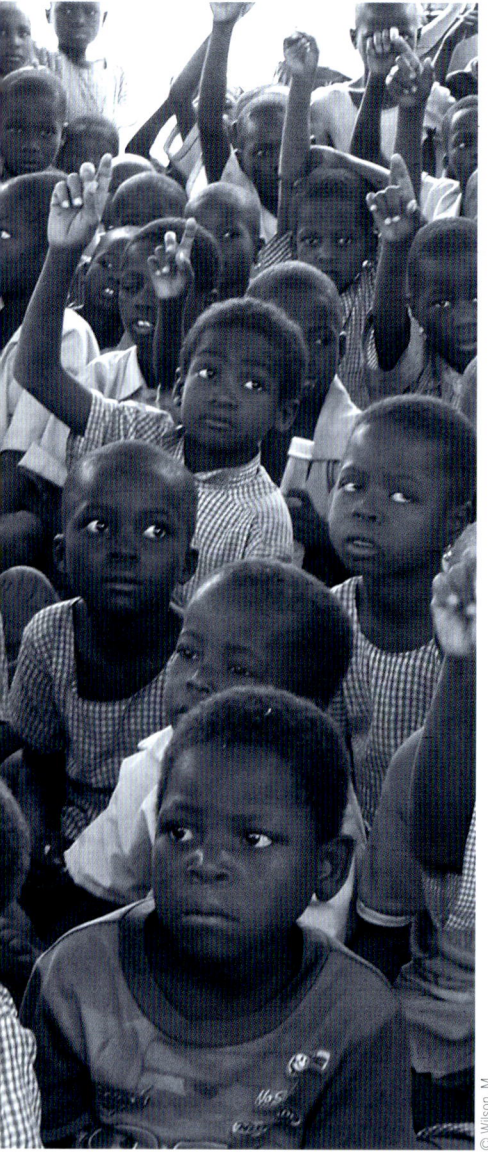

Children confirming haematuria (blood-urine) by show of hands during a schistosomiasis (bilharziasis) education session at a primary school in Bongo, Ghana. Schistosomiasis causes anaemia, stunting and a reduced ability to learn among children.

REFERENCES

1. Gryseels B et al. Human schistosomiasis. *Lancet*, 2006, 368:1006–1018.

2. Steinmann P et al. Schistosomiasis and water resources development: systematic review, meta-analysis, and estimates of people at risk. *Lancet Infectious Diseases*, 2006, 6:411–425.

3. Talla I et al. Outbreak of intestinal schistosomiasis in the Senegal River Basin [in English]. *Annales de la Société Belge de Médecine Tropicale*, 1990, 70:173–180.

4. Chitsulo L et al. The global status of schistosomiasis and its control. *Acta Tropica*, 2000, 77:41–51.

5. Wang LD et al. A strategy to control transmission of *Schistosoma japonicum* in China. *New England Journal of Medicine*, 2009, 360:121–128.

6. Sinuon M et al. Control of *Schistosoma mekongi* in Cambodia: results of eight years of control activities in the two endemic provinces. *Transactions of the Royal Society of Tropical Medicine and Hygiene*, 2007, 101:34–39.

7. *The global burden of disease: 2004 update*. Geneva, World Health Organization, 2008.

8. King CH, Dickman K, Tisch DJ. Reassessment of the cost of chronic helmintic infection: a meta-analysis of disability-related outcomes in endemic schistosomiasis. *Lancet*, 2005, 365:1561–1569.

9. King CH, Dangerfield-Cha M. The unacknowledged impact of chronic schistosomiasis. *Chronic Illness*, 2008, 4:65–79.

10. Parkin DM. The global burden of urinary bladder cancer. *Scandinavian Journal of Urology and Nephrology*, 2008, 42(Suppl. 218):S12–S20.

11. Kjetland EF et al. Association between genital schistosomiasis and HIV in rural Zimbabwean women. *AIDS*, 2006, 20:593–600.

12. van der Werf MJ et al. Quantification of clinical morbidity associated with schistosome infection in sub-Saharan Africa. *Acta Tropica*, 2003, 86:125–139.

13. Amaral RS et al. An analysis of the impact of the Schistosomiasis Control Programme in Brazil [in English]. *Memórias do Instituto Oswaldo Cruz*, 2006, 101(Suppl. 1):S79–S85.

14. Croce D et al. Cost-effectiveness of a successful schistosomiasis control programme in Cambodia (1995–2006). *Acta Tropica*, 2010, 113:279–284.

15. Brooker S et al. Cost and cost-effectiveness of nationwide school-based helminth control in Uganda. *Health Policy and Planning*, 2008, 23:24–35.

16. Hotez PJ, Fenwick A. Schistosomiasis in Africa: an emerging tragedy in our new global health decade. *PLoS Neglected Tropical Diseases*, 2009, 3(9):e485.

17. Gabrielli AF et al. A combined school- and community-based campaign targeting all school-age children of Burkina Faso against schistosomiasis and soil-transmitted helminthiasis: performance, financial costs and implications for sustainability. *Acta Tropica*, 2006, 99:234–242.

18. Kjetland EF et al. Prevention of gynecologic contact bleeding and genital sandy patches by childhood anti-schistosomal treatment. *American Journal of Tropical Medicine and Hygiene*, 2008, 79:79–83.

19. Allen HE et al. New policies for using anthelmintics in high risk groups. *Trends in Parasitology*, 2002, 18:381–382.

20. *WHO preventive chemotherapy and transmission control databank*. Geneva, World Health Organization, 2010 (http://www.who.int/neglected_diseases/preventive_chemotherapy/databank/en/index.html; accessed July 2010).

5.17 Soil-transmitted helminthiases

Abstract

More than 1 billion people are infected with the species of nematode that cause soil-transmitted helminthiases (STH). The infections and the chronic morbidity they cause persist wherever access to effective sanitation is lacking. Burkina Faso, Cambodia and the Lao People's Democratic Republic have reached the World Health Assembly's target (contained in resolution WHA54.19) of treating at least 75% of school-aged children for the disease by 2010.

Description

The four species of helminth sometimes occur concurrently in the same community, resulting in people being infected with more than one species at a time. Also, infections are acquired from an environment contaminated by the worms' infective stages, and so the species are often considered collectively as if they are a single entity. Consequently STH may be used to mean soil-transmitted helminth, soil-transmitted helminth infection or soil-transmitted helminthiases, without reference to the species involved. Care should be taken to be precise about the use of the abbreviation STH, especially in the context of health, where STH could mean soil-transmitted helminthiases relating, say, to ascariasis, or soil-transmitted helminthiases relating to ascariasis and trichuriasis in the same patient. Each species is responsible for a separate set of signs and symptoms, in fact for a separate disease. Hookworms (*Ancylostoma duodenale* and *Necator americanus*) differ in their biology from the common roundworm (*Ascaris lumbricoides*) and in the diseases they cause. Similarly, whipworm (*Trichuris trichiura*) differs from the others, as does the disease that it causes. The convention of referring to the disease caused by hookworms as "hookworm disease" seems to have arisen because the identification of the species of hookworm on the basis of eggs in stools is unreliable. In this report, the abbreviation STH refers to soil-transmitted helminthiases.

People infected with soil-transmitted helminths pass parasite eggs in their faeces. In areas where there is no latrine system, the soil and water around the village or community becomes contaminated with faeces containing these eggs. The persistence of STH is closely linked to contamination of the environment with the faeces of infected people. The symptoms of soil-transmitted helminth infections are nonspecific and become evident only when the infection is particularly severe. Symptoms include nausea, tiredness, abdominal pain and loss of appetite. These infections aggravate malnutrition and amplify rates of anaemia. They impede children's physical growth and cognitive development, contributing significantly to school absenteeism.

Distribution

Soil-transmitted helminthiases are widely distributed in tropical and subtropical areas (*Figure 5.17.1, Figure 5.17.2*). Worldwide, it has been estimated that more than 1 billion people are infected with these diseases (*1*), of whom more than 300 million suffer from severe morbidity. The estimated number (in millions) of soil-transmitted helminth infections in 2003 is presented in *Table 5.17.1*.

Table 5.17.1 Global estimates of cases of soil-transmitted helminth infections, by type, WHO region and age group, 2003[a]

Type of infection and WHO region	Estimated number of soil-transmitted helminth infections (millions) Age group (years)				
	0–4	5–9	10–14	≥15	Total
Ascariasis					
African	28	28	25	92	173
Americas	8	10	10	56	84
Eastern Mediterranean	3	3	3	14	23
South-East Asia	28	33	30	145	237
Western Pacific	55	69	76	505	705
Total	122	143	144	812	1222
Trichuriasis					
African	26	27	23	66	162
Americas	10	12	12	86	100
Eastern Mediterranean	1	1	1	4	7
South-East Asia	18	20	19	90	147
Western Pacific	30	38	41	268	379
Total	85	98	96	514	795
Hookworm disease					
African	9	18	29	142	198
Americas	1	3	5	41	50
Eastern Mediterranean	0	1	1	8	10
South-East Asia	4	10	16	100	130
Western Pacific	7	18	34	293	352
Total	21	50	85	584	740

[a] Adapted from de Silva NR et al (*2*).

Fig. 5.17.1 Distribution of soil-transmitted helminthiases, worldwide, 2009

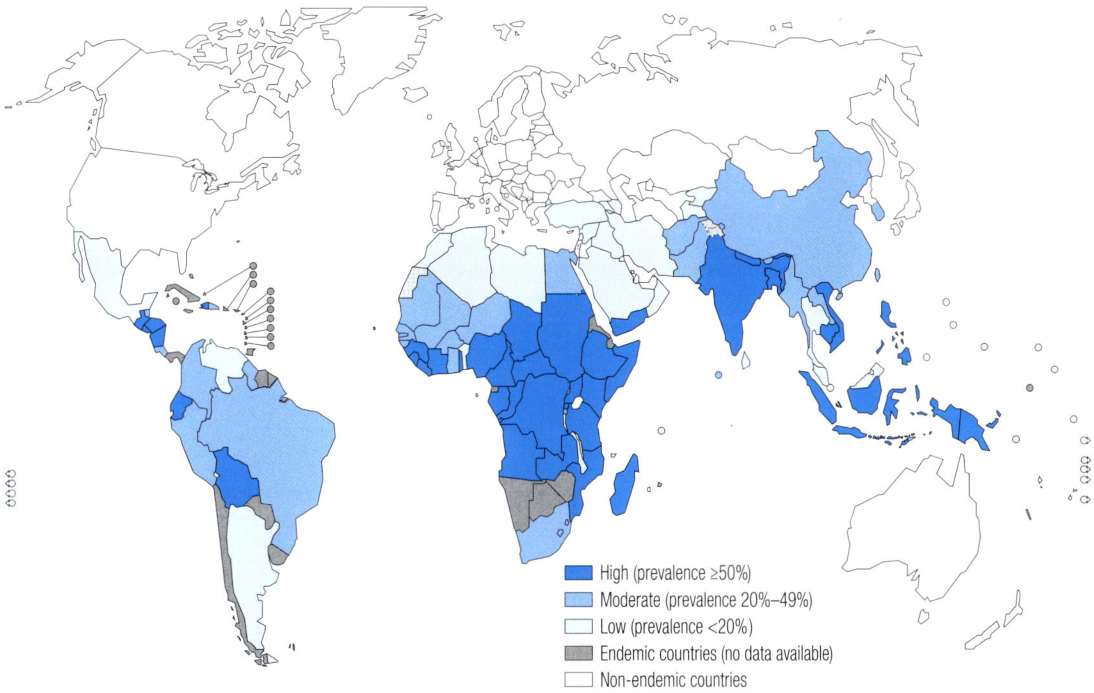

- High (prevalence ≥50%)
- Moderate (prevalence 20%–49%)
- Low (prevalence <20%)
- Endemic countries (no data available)
- Non-endemic countries

Distribution of soil-transmitted helminthiases is focal in many countries. For the detailed epidemiological situation in countries, please refer to *Preventive chemotherapy and transmission control databank*. Geneva, World Health Organization, 2010 (available at: http://www.who.int/neglected_diseases/ preventive_chemotherapy/databank/en/index.html: accessed January 2009).

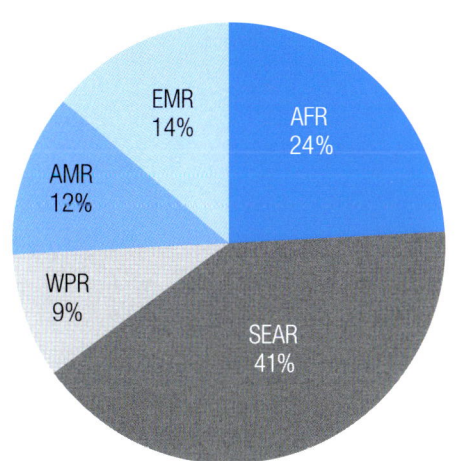

Fig. 5.17.2 Distribution of population requiring preventive chemotherapy for soil-transmitted helminthiases, by WHO region, 2008

- EMR 14%
- AFR 24%
- AMR 12%
- WPR 9%
- SEAR 41%

AFR – African / AMR – The Americas / EMR – Eastern Mediterranean / SEAR – South-East Asia / WPR – Western Pacific

Four countries in the European Region are endemic. The population requiring preventive chemotherapy in these countries is <1% globally and not represented in the chart.

Fig. 5.17.3 Reported coverage of treatment (%) for soil-transmitted helminthiases, by WHO region, 2004–2008

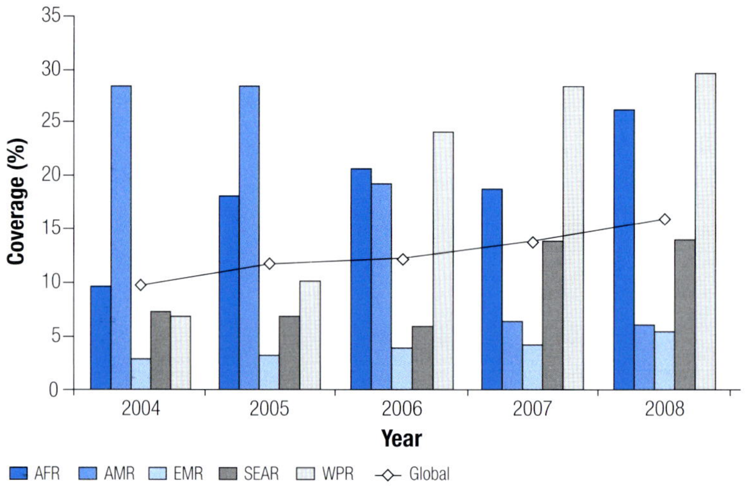

AFR – African / AMR – The Americas / EMR – Eastern Mediterranean / SEAR – South-East Asia / WPR – Western Pacific

Morbidity

The main form of morbidity caused by STH is the negative effect on nutritional status (3). In addition the disease may cause cognitive impairment in children, and complications requiring surgical intervention, such as intestinal and biliary obstructions. Details on the morbidity caused by STH are presented in *Table 5.17.2*.

Table 5.17.2 Morbidity associated with soil-transmitted helminth infections[a]

Type of morbidity	Sign of morbidity	Parasite	Reference
Nutritional impairment	Intestinal bleeding, anaemia	*Ancylostoma duodenale* *Necator americanus*	4
	Malabsorption of nutrients	*Ascaris lumbricoides*	6, 7
	Competition for micronutrients	*Ascaris lumbricoides*	8
	Impaired growth	*Ascaris lumbricoides*	9
	Loss of appetite and reduction of food intake	*Ascaris lumbricoides*	10
	Diarrhoea or dysentery	*Trichuris trichiura*	11
Cognitive impairment	Reduction in fluency and memory	*Trichuris trichiura*	12, 13
Conditions requiring surgical intervention	Intestinal and biliary obstructions	*Ascaris lumbricoides*	5
	Rectal prolapse	*Trichuris trichiura*	14

[a] Adapted from Montresor et al. (*15*).

The prevalence and intensity of infection with *Ascaris* and *Trichuris* typically reach a peak among children aged 5–14 years and subsequently decline among adults. However, although heavy hookworm infections may occur in children, the peak of their prevalence and intensity is commonly reported among those aged 30–44 years or even among people who are older than 50 (*1*). Soil-transmitted helminthiases (especially hookworm) are particularly detrimental to the health of childbearing women and on pregnancy outcomes owing to their impact on nutrition, since they cause iron deficiency and anaemia.

Economic impact

A retrospective study based on data from the Rockefeller Commission evaluated the economic impact of efforts to control hookworm infection in the southern United States; it found that children cured of hookworm were 25% more likely to attend school than untreated children, and having a hookworm-free childhood translated into earning 45% more income during adulthood (*16*). The impact produced by the nutritional and cognitive impairment associated with these infections on the intellectual development and physical fitness of children and adults, and consequently on work capacity and productivity, has been clearly highlighted (*17*).

Prevention and control

Lack of access to safe water and proper sanitation are the main factors in the persistence and prevalence of the disease. During the second half of the 20th century, the progressive improvement in standards of living in North America, Europe and Japan has virtually eliminated STH there. More recently, a similar trend has been observed in emerging economies in Asia, such as Malaysia and the Republic of Korea. The level of sanitation has not significantly improved in the least-developed countries where these infections continue to cause significant morbidity.

Control programmes in endemic countries have demonstrated that the benefits of regular deworming are not limited to reducing direct morbidity. School attendance, school results and productivity improve. An efficient way to reach preschool-aged children for deworming treatment is to integrate this treatment into vaccination campaigns organized for this age group. The inclusion of deworming along with vaccination increases the coverage of the campaign. More than 104 million preschool-aged children (20% of those in need of regular treatment) are dewormed through vaccination campaigns, and coverage is increasing.

An equally efficient way to reach children of school age is through the school system. Countries with few resources but with strong political commitment (for example, Burkina Faso, Cambodia and the Lao People's Democratic Republic) have achieved the target set by the World Health Assembly of treating 75% of school-aged children by using schools as treatment centres.

Approximately 16% of school-aged children in need of regular treatment in endemic countries (100 million children) receive periodic treatment. Recent estimates report that it would cost US$ 33 000 to cover 1 million schoolchildren (*18*). Despite the growth in coverage rates, the target of 75% coverage of the world's school-age children will not be reached unless implementation increases significantly in order to take account of current needs and demographic growth. (*Figure 5.17.3*).

Another important aspect to be considered is that one third of school-aged children receive anthelminthic medicine through the Global Programme to Eliminate Lymphatic Filariasis, which distributes albendazole together with ivermectin or diethylcarbamazine. Once this programme eliminates lymphatic filariasis in a community (normally after 6 years of mass distribution of medicine), treatment at the population level is generally discontinued. Mechanisms to maintain the anthelminthic distribution of benzimidazoles (albendazole or mebendazole) after the Global Programme to Eliminate Lymphatic Filariasis ceases operating should be put in place so the advantages obtained by the programme in controlling STH are not lost.

Assessment

Many countries where soil-transmitted helminthiases are endemic will not attain the target set for 2010 by World Health Assembly resolution WHA54.19, and adopted in 2001, to treat at least 75% of school-aged children. In 2008, 16% of infected children were treated worldwide. In 2008, the Global Programme to Eliminate Lymphatic Filariasis distributed albendazole as part of its treatment for lymphatic filariasis, thereby providing treatment for soil-transmitted helminthiases to 65 million children. There will be a significant shortfall in access to medicine when this programme ends.

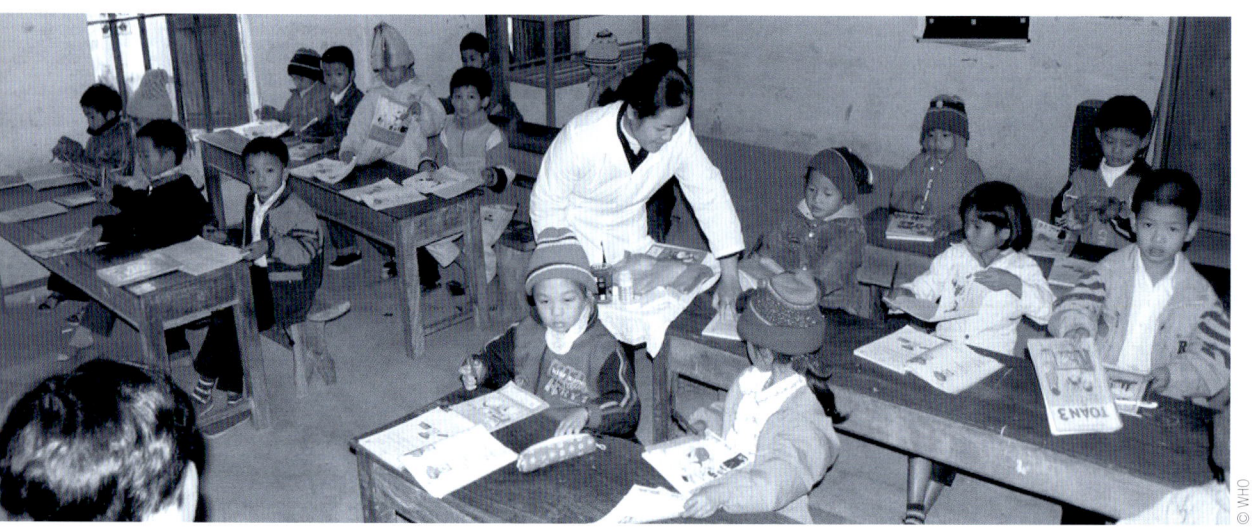

Distribution of mebendazole to school children in Bac Can province in Viet Nam. The use of the school infrastructure to deliver deworming allows a low-cost distribution of drugs and ensures a higher rate of treatment.

REFERENCES

1. Hotez PJ et al. Rescuing the bottom billion through control of neglected tropical diseases. *Lancet*, 2009, 373:1570–1575.
2. de Silva NR et al. Soil-transmitted helminth infections: updating the global picture. *Trends in Parasitology*, 2003, 19:547–551.
3. Hall A et al. A review and meta-analysis of the impact of intestinal worms on child growth and nutrition. *Maternal and Child Nutrition*, 2008, 4(Suppl. 1):S118–S236.
4. Stoltzfus RJ et al. Hemoquant determination of hookworm-related blood loss and its role in iron deficiency in African children. *American Journal of Tropical Medicine and Hygiene*, 1996, 55:399–404.
5. de Silva NR, Chan MS, Bundy DA. Morbidity and mortality due to ascariasis: re-estimation and sensitivity analysis of global numbers at risk. *Tropical Medicine and International Health*, 1997, 2:519–528.
6. Solomons NW. Pathways to the impairment of human nutritional status by gastrointestinal pathogens. *Parasitology*, 1993, 107(Suppl.):S19–S35.
7. Crompton DWT, Nesheim MC. Nutritional impact of intestinal helminthiasis during the human life cycle. *Annual Review of Nutrition*, 2002, 22:35–59.
8. Curtale F et al. Intestinal helminths and risk of anaemia among Nepalese children. *Panminerva Medica*, 1993, 35:159–166.
9. Taren DL et al. Contributions of ascariasis to poor nutritional status in children from Chiriqui Province, Republic of Panama. *Parasitology*, 1987, 95:603–613.
10. Stephenson LS et al. Physical fitness, growth and appetite of Kenyan school boys with hookworm, *Trichuris trichiura* and *Ascaris lumbricoides* infections are improved four months after a single dose of albendazole. *Journal of Nutrition*, 1993, 123:1036–1046.
11. Callender JE et al. Growth and development four years after treatment for the Trichuris dysentery syndrome. *Acta Paediatrica*, 1998, 87:1247–1249.
12. Nokes C et al. Parasitic helminth infection and cognitive function in school children. *Proceedings of the Royal Society B: Biological Sciences*, 1992, 247:77–81.
13. Kvalsvig JD, Cooppan RM, Connolly KJ. The effects of parasite infections on cognitive processes in children. *Annals of Tropical Medicine and Parasitology*, 1991, 85:551–568.
14. *Intestinal protozoan and helminthic infections. Report of a WHO Scientific Group.* Geneva, World Health Organization, 1981.
15. Montresor A et al. *Helminth control in school age children: a guide for managers of control programmes.* Geneva, World Health Organization, 2002.
16. McGuire RA, Elman C. *The prevalence of parasitic intestinal worms in the early twentieth-century American south and their demographic and economic correlates* [working paper]. Akron, OH, University of Akron, 2003.
17. Guyatt H. Do intestinal nematodes affect productivity in adulthood? *Parasitology Today*, 2000, 16:153–158.
18. Montresor A et al. Estimation of the cost of large-scale school deworming programmes with benzimidazoles. *Transactions of the Royal Society of Tropical Medicine and Hygiene*, 2010, 104:129–132.

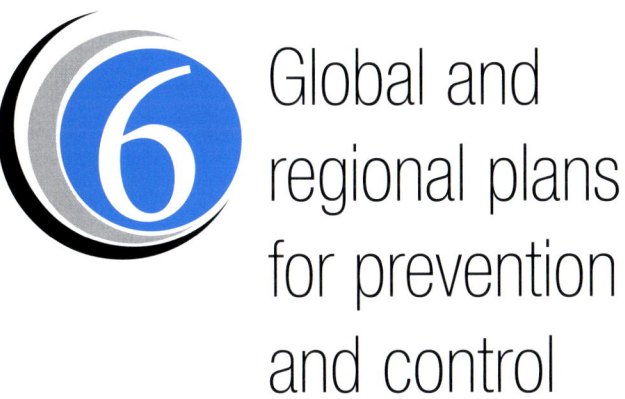
6 Global and regional plans for prevention and control

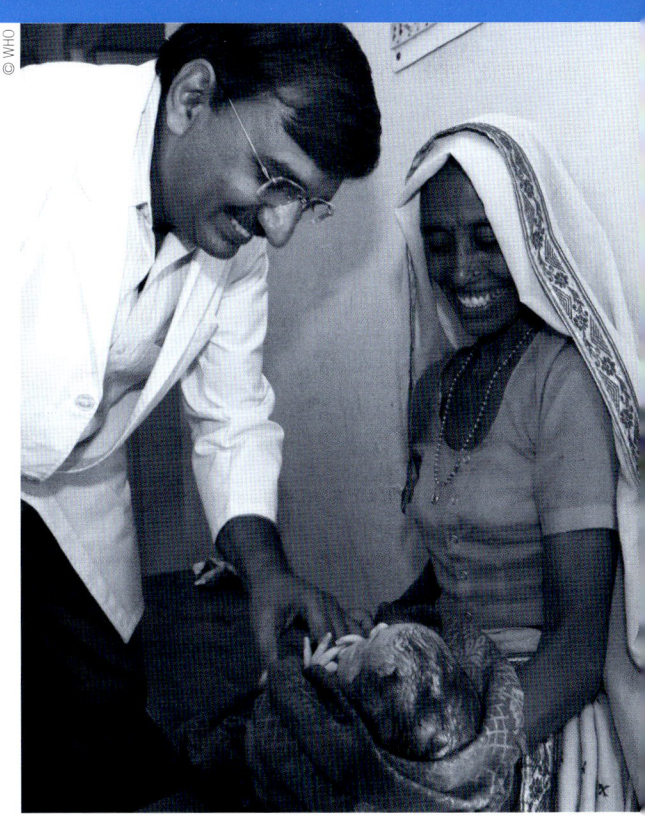

6.1 Health targets

The *Global plan to combat neglected tropical diseases 2008–2015* (*1*) was prepared by WHO after deliberations among technical staff at headquarters and regional offices, country representatives and their staff, and external experts. In keeping with the Millennium Development Goals, the global plan aims to prevent, control, eliminate or eradicate NTDs. The targets for the plan's period are:

> to eliminate or eradicate those diseases targeted in resolutions of the World Health Assembly and WHO's regional committees;

> to reduce significantly the burden of other diseases for which interventions exist;

> to ensure that novel approaches to treatment are available, promoted and accessible for diseases that have few treatments or control strategies.

Each of the nine strategic areas of the global plan proposes a series of actions to meet specific targets during 2008–2015. The strategic areas for action are:

1. to assess the burden of NTDs including zoonoses;
2. to develop integrated approaches and multi-intervention packages for disease control;
3. to strengthen health-care systems and capacity building;
4. to formulate evidence for advocacy to promote prevention, treatment and control;
5. to ensure free and timely access to high-quality medicines and diagnostic and preventive tools;
6. to improve access to innovation;
7. to strengthen the integration of vector management and veterinary public-health interventions at the human–animal health interface;
8. to consolidate partnerships and mobilize resources;
9. to promote an intersectoral, interprogrammatic approach to NTD control.

Since the list of NTDs presented in this report is not exhaustive, and has regional and national variations, diseases need to be prioritized for action and appropriate strategies should be developed for control. Some diseases can be controlled with a multi-intervention package implemented on a large scale, while others require taking intensified actions in focus areas.

WHO's regional offices have developed individual action plans to combat NTDs, and each plan focuses on regionally prioritized diseases. Regional specificities and priorities for prevention and control of NTDs are set out below (*Table 6.1.1*). There is no report from the European Region since NTDs have little direct public-health effect on its countries, but the region should be mindful of the opportunities for infections to travel as evidenced by the arrival of Chagas disease in southern Europe (see section 5.7).

Table 6.1.1 Neglected tropical diseases given priority for prevention and control, by WHO region and source of document

WHO region and source	Priority diseases
African Region AFRO workplan 2006–2007 (DDC/CPC)	Buruli ulcer Dracunculiasis Human African trypanosomiasis Leishmaniasis Leprosy Lymphatic filariasis Loiasis Onchocerciasis Schistosomiasis Soil-transmitted helminthiases
Eastern Mediterranean Region EMRO NTD control inter-country workplan 2006–2007	Dracunculiasis Human African trypanosomiasis Leishmaniasis Leprosy Lymphatic filariasis Schistosomiasis and intestinal parasitic infections Zoonotic cutaneous leishmaniasis Zoonotic diseases (brucellosis, rabies, hydatidosis)
Region of the Americas Regional strategic framework for prevention and control of neglected diseases in neglected populations in Latin America and the Caribbean 2006–2020	Chagas disease Dengue Echinococcosis (hydatidosis) Fascioliasis Hookworm disease Leishmaniasis Leprosy Lymphatic filariasis Onchocerciasis Other soil-transmitted infections Schistosomiasis *Taeniasis solium* and cysticercosis Trachoma Rabies
South-East Asia Region SEARO workplan 2006–2007 (communicable disease prevention and control)	Dengue and dengue haemorrhagic fever Rabies Soil-transmitted helminthiases Japanese encephalitis Leishmaniasis Leprosy Lymphatic filariasis Trachoma and leptospirosis Yaws
Western Pacific Region WPRO workplan 2006–2007	Malaria and other vector-borne and parasitic diseases in Cambodia Dengue and dengue haemorrhagic fever Foodborne trematodiasis Leprosy Lymphatic filariasis Schistosomiasis Soil-transmitted helminthiases Rabies and zoonoses

6.2 Regional plans

WHO's regional offices and the Member States they support have responded to the global plan by developing regional plans to identify how NTDs can be prevented and controlled in their regions. Copies of the regional plans from the African, Americas, Eastern Mediterranean and South-East Asia regions have been published in electronic format and are attached to this report. The report from the Western Pacific Region, which has also been published electronically, is concerned only with the prevention and control of dengue fever and dengue haemorrhagic fever.

REFERENCE

1. *Global plan to combat neglected tropical diseases 2008–2015.* Geneva, World Health Organization, 2007 (WHO/CDS/NTD/2007.3).

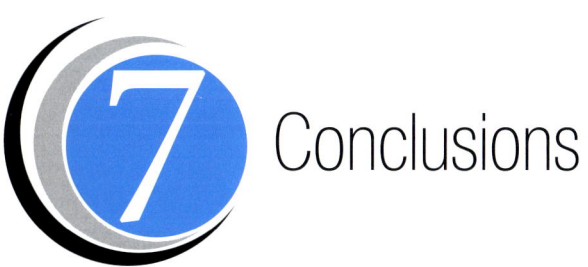
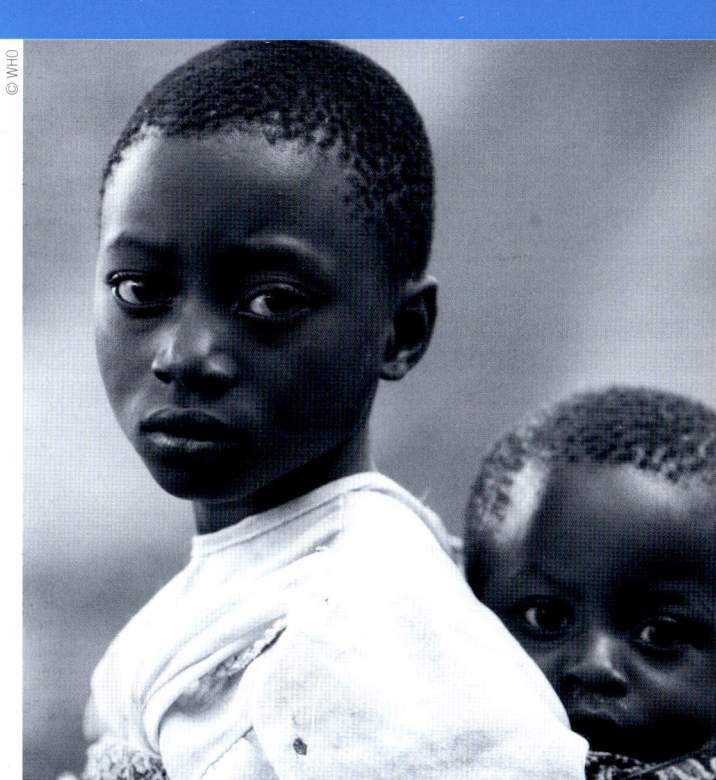

7 Conclusions

This report is the first of its kind to detail the work of WHO and its partners in overcoming the global impact of neglected tropical diseases, work that began during the early years of WHO. The report contains quantitative information and evidence about the global situation of NTDs in the world today, focusing on progress made in overcoming the transmission of widely prevalent pathogens and their associated morbidity and mortality in millions of people. Although NTDs are a diverse group of diseases, they share in common a stranglehold on populations whose lives are ravaged by poverty. During the past decade, the wider international community has recognized that this situation is unacceptable, and this recognition has stimulated the growth of a community of partners committed to bringing resources and expertise to the task of overcoming NTDs.

WHO provides technical advice to governments and other organizations, develops strategies for prevention and control, compiles quantitative information about the distribution of NTDs and the coverage and implementation of activities, and coordinates the work of its community of partners.

Evidence provided throughout this report demonstrates that steady progress is being made. The effort is directed towards achieving the targets for NTD control set by the World Health Assembly that will in turn contribute to attaining the Millennium Development Goals. Improvements in health will surely have a major beneficial impact on development. Onchocerciasis has declined in west Africa and is being tackled in the rest of the continent. The prevalence of leprosy worldwide has declined steadily. Schistosomiasis has been defeated in China. Dracunculiasis should soon be eradicated. New public-health approaches for controlling NTDs in communities have been developed and are being implemented. Processes are being strengthened to facilitate assessment of the quality of medicines and procurement management. A Strategic and Technical Advisory Group for NTDs, reporting to WHO's Director-General, has been established and has begun work. Millions of people are now receiving treatment free of charge with safety-tested medicines of assured quality. Many health workers in endemic countries have been trained in aspects of NTD control, thereby strengthening national health systems.

We should not get carried away with success. Many challenges need attention and action. Millions more people are in need of free treatment with high-quality medicines. Millions more need care and treatment for rabies, echinococcosis, leishmaniasis and other seemingly intractable NTDs. Drug resistance may emerge as control interventions based on the distribution of medicines expand. Vector control must be increased and coordinated, in many cases with water supply and water development projects. In the long term, economic growth and stability will eventually ensure that safe water and sanitation are provided for all peoples: a prerequisite for banishing NTDs from the human experience.

In April 2007, Dr Margaret Chan, WHO's Director-General, addressed the NTD partners. She set out her vision for the future of NTD control and concluded: "For the first time, we have a head start on these ancient companions of poverty. For the first time, more than 1 billion people left behind by socioeconomic progress have a chance to catch up. I believe this is our shared ambition".

Overcoming neglected tropical diseases: 7 gains, 7 challenges

Gains

1. **Recognition of the importance of global control of neglected tropical diseases.** A more reliable evaluation of the significance of NTDs in terms of their impact on public health and economies has stimulated new thinking in public health, leading to the adoption of five strategic approaches for widespread interventions. This evaluation has convinced governments, donors, the pharmaceutical industry and other agencies, including NGOs, to invest in NTD prevention and control.

2. **Progress in prevention and control of neglected tropical diseases.** Prevention and control activities for NTDs have been included in the policies and budgets of many endemic countries. This has led to the development of interventions appropriate to existing health systems, often with the support of implementing partners.

3. **Increased commitment.** The development of plans by WHO's regional offices in response to the *Global plan to combat neglected tropical diseases 2008–2015* (*1*) has led to growing awareness of NTDs and the suffering they cause.

4. **Successful outcomes.** Global efforts to control "hidden" diseases, such as dracunculiasis, leprosy, lymphatic filariasis and yaws, have yielded progressive gains including the imminent eradication of dracunculiasis.

5. **Regional success.** Achievements in the control of Chagas disease, human African trypanosomiasis, onchocerciasis, schistosomiasis and trachoma have generated greater awareness and wider recognition of the disease burden that affects poor people.

6. **Engagement with the pharmaceutical industry.** Involvement of the industry with NTDs and their subsequent donations to support control efforts have increased access to high-quality medicines free of charge for hundreds of millions of poor people (*Table 7.1*).

7. **Expanded collaboration between partners.** The increasing willingness and commitment of local and global communities of partners to work with endemic countries have brought resources, innovation, expertise and advocacy to efforts to overcome NTDs. Intersectoral collaboration involving education, nutrition and agriculture has reinforced NTD control efforts (*2*).

Table 7.1 Major donations of medicines for controlling neglected tropical diseases made by the pharmaceutical industry

Medicine	Donation
Albendazole	Unlimited supply for as long as needed from GlaxoSmithKline for lymphatic filariasis; donation made through WHO
Azithromycin	Unlimited quantity from Pfizer in the context of SAFE
Eflornithine	Unlimited quantity until 2012 from sanofi-aventis for human African trypanosomiasis; donation made through WHO
Ivermectin	Unlimited supply for as long as needed donated directly to countries by Merck & Co., Inc., for lymphatic filariasis and onchocerciasis
Multidrug therapy (rifampicin, clofazimine and dapsone in blister packs) and loose clofazimine	Unlimited supply for as long as needed for leprosy and its complications from Novartis; donation made through WHO
Mebendazole	50 million tablets annually from Johnson & Johnson for soil-transmitted helminthiases control programmes for children. From 2011, this will increase to 200 million annually
Melarsoprol	Unlimited quantity until 2012 from sanofi-aventis for human African trypanosomiasis; donation made through WHO
Nifurtimox	900 000 tablets (120 mg) per year by 2014 from Bayer for treatment of Chagas disease and human African trypanosomiasis; donation made through WHO
Pentamidine	Unlimited quantity by 2012 from sanofi-aventis for human African trypanosomiasis; donation made through WHO
Praziquantel	200 million tablets during 2008–2017 from Merck KGaA for schistosomiasis; donation made through WHO
Suramin	Unlimited quantity by 2012 from Bayer for human African trypanosomiasis; donation made through WHO
Triclabendazole	From Novartis for fascioliasis; donation made through WHO

Challenges

1. **Commitment of resources.** Despite global economic constraints, support from the United States, the United Kingdom, Spain, other countries, agencies and NGOs will need to be sustained, and this should encourage others to expand their support for developing the services needed to overcome NTDs.

2. **Declining relevant expertise.** Expertise in individual NTDs is lacking in some countries or continues to decline. The decline is most severe in vector control, case-management, pesticide management and veterinary aspects of public health. As expansion of prevention and control activities in endemic countries increases, the need will increase to strengthen health systems, and to train and support staff with technical and management expertise.

3. **Expanding use of preventive chemotherapy.** Targets for coverage set by the World Health Assembly for control of lymphatic filariasis, schistosomiasis, soil-transmitted helminthiases and trachoma will not be met, especially in the African and South-East Asia regions, unless interventions with preventive chemotherapy increase.

4. **Insufficient quantities of quality-assured medicines for neglected tropical diseases.** Donations of praziquantel from the private sector and funds for its production are insufficient to meet the quantities of this essential medicine needed to control schistosomiasis. For lymphatic filariasis, two of the three medicines required (albendazole and ivermectin) are donated. The third (diethylcarbamazine citrate [DEC]) needs to be purchased. The provision of medicines to treat soil-transmitted helminthiases needs also to be increased significantly. Production of medicines for NTDs needs to become attractive to manufacturers of generic drugs.

5. **Targeted research for neglected tropical diseases.** A research strategy is required to develop and introduce new medicines, notably for leishmaniasis and trypanosomiasis; new methods for vector control; vaccines for dengue; and new diagnostics that will be accessible to all who need them.

6. **Improved quantitative information systems.** As control interventions reach more people and new technologies are embraced, quicker responses will need to be made to information about the epidemiology, transmission and burden of NTDs. Similarly, programme managers will need to react quickly to information about the coverage, compliance, acceptance and impact of interventions.

7. **Global changes.** Planning for the development of prevention and control measures for NTDs should take into account the possible effects of porous borders, population growth and migration, the movements of livestock and vectors, and the political and geographical consequences of climate change.

REFERENCES

1. *Global plan to combat neglected tropical diseases 2008–2015.* Geneva, World Health Organization, 2007 (WHO/CDS/NTD/2007.3).
2. *Report of the global partners' meeting on neglected tropical diseases.* Geneva, World Health Organization, 2007 (WHO/CDS/NTD/2007.4).

Annexes

Annex 1. Resolutions of the World Health Assembly (WHA) on neglected tropical diseases

Disease	WHA resolution number	Title	Year
Vector-borne disease	WHA1.12	Vector biology and control	1948
Vector-borne disease	WHA2.18	Expert Committee on insecticides: report on the first session	1949
Endemic treponematoses	WHA2.36	Bejel and other treponematoses	1949
Leprosy	WHA2.43	Leprosy	1949
Rabies	WHA3.20	Rabies	1950
Trachoma	WHA3.22	Trachoma	1950
Hydatidosis	WHA3.23	Hydatidosis	1950
Schistosomiasis and soil-transmitted helminthiases	WHA3.26	Bilharziasis	1950
Vector-borne disease	WHA3.43	Labelling and distribution of insecticides	1950
Trachoma	WHA4.29	Trachoma	1951
Vector-borne disease	WHA4.30	Supply of insecticides	1951
Leprosy	WHA5.28	Leprosy	1952
Vector-borne disease	WHA5.29	Supply and requirements of insecticides: world position	1952
Leprosy	WHA6.19	Expert Committee on leprosy: first report	1953
Leprosy	WHA9.45	Inter-regional conference on leprosy control, 1958	1956
Vector-borne disease	WHA13.54	Vector-borne diseases and malaria eradication	1960
Vector-borne disease	WHA22.40	Research on methods of vector control	1969
Vector-borne disease	WHA23.33	Research on alternative methods of vector control	1970
Research	WHA27.52	Intensification of research on tropical parasitic diseases	1974
Leprosy	WHA27.58	Coordination and strengthening of leprosy control	1974
Schistosomiasis	WHA28.53	Schistosomiasis	1975
Avoidable blindness (for both onchocerciasis and trachoma)	WHA28.54	Prevention of blindness	1975
Leprosy	WHA28.56	Leprosy control	1975
Research	WHA28.71	WHO's role in the development and coordination of research in tropical diseases	1975

Disease	WHA resolution number	Title	Year
Schistosomiasis	WHA29.58	Schistosomiasis	1976
Leprosy	WHA29.70	Leprosy control	1976
Leprosy	WHA30.36	Leprosy control	1977
Research	WHA30.42	Special Programme for Research and Training in Tropical Diseases	1977
Zoonoses	WHA31.48	Prevention and control of zoonoses and foodborne diseases due to animal products	1978
Endemic treponematoses	WHA31.58	Control of endemic treponematoses	1978
Leprosy	WHA32.39	Leprosy	1979
Dracunculiasis	WHA34.25	International drinking-water supply and sanitation decade	1981
Human African trypanosomiasis	WHA36.31	African human trypanosomiasis	1983
Dracunculiasis	WHA39.21	Elimination of dracunculiasis	1986
Leprosy	WHA40.35	Towards the elimination of leprosy	1987
Dracunculiasis	WHA42.25	International Drinking Water Supply and Sanitation Decade	1989
Dracunculiasis	WHA42.29	Elimination of dracunculiasis	1989
Vector-borne disease	WHA42.31	Control of disease vectors and pests	1989
Research	WHA43.18	Tropical disease research	1990
Dracunculiasis	WHA44.5	Eradication of dracunculiasis	1991
Leprosy	WHA44.9	Leprosy	1991
Dengue and dengue haemorrhagic fever	WHA46.31	Dengue prevention and control	1993
Onchocerciasis	WHA47.32	Onchocerciasis control through ivermectin distribution	1994
Vector-borne disease	WHA50.13	Promotion of chemical safety, with special attention to persistent organic pollutants	1997
Lymphatic filariasis	WHA50.29	Elimination of lymphatic filariasis as a public health problem	1997
Dracunculiasis	WHA50.35	Eradication of dracunculiasis	1997
Human African trypanosomiasis	WHA50.36	African trypanosomiasis	1997
Trachoma	WHA51.11	Global elimination of blinding trachoma	1998
Chagas disease	WHA51.14	Elimination of transmission of Chagas disease	1998
Leprosy	WHA51.15	Elimination of leprosy as a public health problem	1998

Disease	WHA resolution number	Title	Year
Schistosomiasis and soil-transmitted helminthiases	WHA54.19	Schistosomiasis and soil-transmitted helminth infections	2001
Dengue and dengue haemorrhagic fever	WHA55.17	Prevention and control of dengue fever and dengue haemorrhagic fever	2002
Human African trypanosomiasis	WHA56.7	Pan African tsetse and trypanosomiasis eradication campaign	2003
Avoidable blindness (for both onchocerciasis and trachoma)	WHA56.26	Elimination of avoidable blindness	2003
Buruli ulcer	WHA57.1	Surveillance and control of *Mycobacterium ulcerans* disease (Buruli ulcer)	2004
Human African trypanosomiasis	WHA57.2	Control of human African trypanosomiasis	2004
Dracunculiasis	WHA57.9	Eradication of dracunculiasis	2004
Avoidable blindness (for both onchocerciasis and trachoma)	WHA59.25	Prevention of avoidable blindness and visual impairment	2006
Leishmaniasis	WHA60.13	Control of leishmaniasis	2007
Avoidable blindness (for both onchocerciasis and trachoma)	WHA62.1	Prevention of avoidable blindness and visual impairment	2009
Chagas disease	WHA63.20	Chagas disease: control and elimination	2010

Annex 2. Official list of indicators for monitoring progress on the Millennium Development Goals

Millennium Development Goals (MDGs)	
Goals and targets from the Millennium Declaration	**Indicators for monitoring progress**
Goal 1: Eradicate extreme poverty and hunger	
Target 1.A: Halve, between 1990 and 2015, the proportion of people whose income is less than one dollar a day	1.1 Proportion of population living on less than US$ 1 (PPP) per day[a] 1.2 Poverty gap ratio 1.3 Share of poorest quintile in national consumption
Target 1.B: Achieve full and productive employment and decent work for all, including women and young people	1.4 Growth rate of gross domestic product per person employed 1.5 Employment-to-population ratio 1.6 Proportion of employed people living on less than US$ 1 (PPP) per day 1.7 Proportion of own-account and contributing family workers in total employment
Target 1.C: Halve, between 1990 and 2015, the proportion of people who suffer from hunger	1.8 Prevalence of underweight children aged less than 5 years 1.9 Proportion of population below minimum level of dietary energy consumption
Goal 2: Achieve universal primary education	
Target 2.A: Ensure that, by 2015, children everywhere, boys and girls alike, will be able to complete a full course of primary schooling	2.1 Net enrolment ratio in primary education 2.2 Proportion of pupils starting grade 1 who reach last grade of primary school 2.3 Literacy rate of 15–24 year-olds, women and men
Goal 3: Promote gender equality and empower women	
Target 3.A: Eliminate gender disparity in primary and secondary education, preferably by 2005, and in all levels of education no later than 2015	3.1 Ratios of girls to boys in primary, secondary and tertiary education 3.2 Share of women in wage employment in the nonagricultural sector 3.3 Proportion of seats held by women in national parliament
Goal 4: Reduce child mortality	
Target 4.A: Reduce by two thirds, between 1990 and 2015, the under-five mortality rate	4.1 Under-five mortality rate 4.2 Infant mortality rate 4.3 Proportion of 1-year-old children immunized against measles
Goal 5: Improve maternal health	
Target 5.A: Reduce by three quarters, between 1990 and 2015, the maternal mortality ratio	5.1 Maternal mortality ratio 5.2 Proportion of births attended by skilled health personnel
Target 5.B: Achieve, by 2015, universal access to reproductive health care	5.3 Contraceptive prevalence rate 5.4 Adolescent birth rate 5.5 Antenatal care coverage (at least one visit and at least four visits) 5.6 Unmet need for family planning

Goal 6: Combat HIV/AIDS, malaria and other diseases

Target 6.A: Have halted by 2015 and begun to reverse the spread of HIV/AIDS	6.1 HIV prevalence among population aged 15–24 years 6.2 Condom use at last high-risk sex 6.3 Proportion of population aged 15–24 years with comprehensive correct knowledge of HIV/AIDS 6.4 Ratio of school attendance of orphans to school attendance of non-orphans aged 10–14 years
Target 6.B: Achieve, by 2010, universal access to treatment for HIV/AIDS for all those who need it	6.5 Proportion of population with advanced HIV infection who have access to antiretroviral drugs
Target 6.C: Have halted by 2015 and begun to reverse the incidence of malaria and other major diseases	6.6 Incidence and death rates associated with malaria 6.7 Proportion of children aged less than 5 years sleeping under insecticide-treated bednets 6.8 Proportion of children aged less than 5 years with fever who are treated with appropriate antimalarial drugs 6.9 Incidence, prevalence and death rates associated with tuberculosis 6.10 Proportion of tuberculosis cases detected and cured under directly observed treatment, short course

Goal 7: Ensure environmental sustainability

Target 7.A: Integrate the principles of sustainable development into a countries' policies and programmes, and reverse the loss of environmental resources	7.1 Proportion of land area covered by forest 7.2 CO_2 emissions, total, per capita and per US$ 1 GDP (PPP) 7.3 Consumption of ozone-depleting substances 7.4 Proportion of fish stocks within safe biological limits
Target 7.B: Reduce biodiversity loss, achieving, by 2010, a significant reduction in the rate of loss	7.5 Proportion of total water resources used 7.6 Proportion of terrestrial and marine areas protected 7.7 Proportion of species threatened with extinction
Target 7.C: Halve, by 2015, the proportion of people without sustainable access to safe drinking-water and basic sanitation	7.8 Proportion of population using an improved drinking water source 7.9 Proportion of population using an improved sanitation facility
Target 7.D: By 2020, to have achieved a significant improvement in the lives of at least 100 million slum dwellers	7.10 Proportion of urban population living in slums[b]

Goal 8: Develop a global partnership for development

Target 8.A: Develop further an open, rule-based, predictable, nondiscriminatory trading and financial system Includes a commitment to good governance, development and poverty reduction, nationally and internationally Target 8.B: Address the special needs of the least developed countries Includes tariff-free and quota-free access for exports from the least-developed countries; an enhanced programme of debt relief for heavily indebted poor countries and cancellation of official bilateral debt; and more generous official development assistance for countries committed to poverty reduction	Some of the indicators listed below are monitored separately for the least-developed countries, Africa, landlocked developing countries and small island developing states Official development assistance 8.1 Net official development assistance, total and to the least developed countries, as percentage of OECD/DAC donors' gross national income 8.2 Proportion of total bilateral, sector-allocable official development assistance of OECD/DAC donors to basic social services (basic education, primary health care, nutrition, safe water and sanitation) 8.3 Proportion of bilateral official development assistance of OECD/DAC donors that is untied 8.4 Official development assistance received in landlocked developing countries as a proportion of their gross national incomes 8.5 Official development assistance received in small island developing states as a proportion of their gross national incomes

Target 8.C: Address the special needs of landlocked developing countries and small island developing states (through the Programme of Action for the Sustainable Development of Small Island Developing States and the outcome of the twenty-second special session of the General Assembly)	Market access	
	8.1	Proportion of total developed country imports (by value and excluding arms) from developing countries and least-developed countries, admitted free of duty
	8.2	Average tariffs imposed by developed countries on agricultural products, textiles and clothing from developing countries
	8.3	Agricultural support estimate for OECD countries as a percentage of their gross domestic product
	8.4	Proportion of official development assistance provided to help build trade capacity
Target 8.D: Deal comprehensively with the debt problems of developing countries through national and international measures in order to make debt sustainable in the long term	Debt sustainability	
	8.5	Total number of countries that have reached their HIPC decision points and number that have reached their heavily indebted poor countries completion points (cumulative)
	8.6	Debt relief committed under heavily indebted poor countries and MDRI initiatives
	8.7	Debt service as a percentage of exports of goods and services
Target 8.E: In cooperation with pharmaceutical companies, provide access to affordable essential drugs in developing countries	8.8	Proportion of population with access to affordable essential drugs on a sustainable basis
Target 8.F: In cooperation with the private sector, make available the benefits of new technologies, especially information and communications	8.9	Telephone lines/100 population
	8.10	Cellular subscribers/100 population
	8.11	Internet users/100 population

The Millennium Development Goals and targets come from the Millennium Declaration, signed by 189 countries, including 147 heads of state and government, in September 2000 (http://www.un.org/millennium/declaration/ares552e.htm) and from further agreement by Member States at the 2005 World Summit (Resolution adopted by the General Assembly, A/RES/60/1, http://www.un.org/Docs/journal/asp/ws.asp?m=A/RES/60/1). The goals and targets are interrelated and should be seen as a whole. They represent a partnership between developed countries and developing countries "to create an environment – at the national and global levels alike – which is conducive to development and the elimination of poverty".

---

[a] To monitor poverty trends in countries, indicators based on national poverty lines should be used where available.

[b] The actual proportion of people living in slums is measured by a proxy, represented by the urban population living in households with at least one of the following four characteristics: (a) lack of access to improved water supply; (b) lack of access to improved sanitation; (c) overcrowding (3 or more people per room); and (d) dwellings made of non-durable material.

Annex 3. Summary of metadata (*1*) with relevant code or codes from the *International statistical classification of diseases and related health problems*, 10th revision (*2*)

5.1 Dengue and other arboviral diseases (A90, A91)	
Global number of cases reported	Dengue and other mosquito-borne viral fevers (A90, A91, A92)

5.2 Rabies (A82.0, A82.1)	
Risk categories for rabies are defined based on the likelihood of contracting human rabies in a given country or area	No risk: countries or areas that are considered rabies-free (human and animal rabies historically not reported and/or not reported by surveillance in any animal species, domestic or wild)
	Low risk: countries or areas with no dog-to-dog rabies transmission (because of dog control or elimination operations or because these areas were historically free of rabies in dogs) but with wildlife (wild-carnivore mediated and/or bat-mediated) rabies. Throughout these areas, human rabies biologics (vaccines and immunoglobulin) and expertise to provide post-exposure prophylaxis are readily available
	Moderate risk: countries or areas with only sporadic cases of rabies in dogs and wildlife (wild carnivore-mediated and/or bat-mediated). In these areas, human biologics and expertise to provide post-exposure prophylaxis are mostly available in major urban centres
	High risk: countries or areas with sustained dog-to-dog rabies transmission and no or little wildlife rabies (with the exception of the Amazonian forest where rabies in vampire bats is present and represents a high risk for humans). In these countries or areas, access to human biologics and expertise to provide post-exposure prophylaxis are usually very limited

5.3 Trachoma (A71)	
Trachomatous inflammation – follicular (TF)	Trachomatous inflammation – follicular: defined as the presence of at least 5 follicles at least 0.5 mm in diameter in the central part of the upper tarsal conjunctiva (*3*)
Trachomatous inflammation – intense (TI)	Trachomatous inflammation – intense: defined as pronounced inflammatory thickening of the upper tarsal conjunctiva obscuring more than half the normal deep tarsal vessels (*3*)
Endemic	Countries with communities where the prevalence of active trachoma in children aged 1–9 years is greater than 10% or where the prevalence of trichiasis in people aged 15 years or older is 1% and where trachoma elimination activities are required
Non-endemic	Countries not requiring implementation of trachoma elimination activities

5.4 Buruli ulcer (A31.1)

Endemic	A country or territory with ≥1 laboratory-confirmed case of Buruli ulcer
Global number of new cases	Total number of new probable cases of Buruli ulcer diagnosed within the reported year
Mapping	Using routinely reported data from health facilities to identify communities with the disease
Surveillance	Routine monthly reporting of Buruli ulcer data (using standardized form BU02) from peripheral to central levels
BU02 form	Form for reporting data from health facilities to central levels and WHO
Confirmed cases	Buruli ulcer cases that have been confirmed by polymerase chain reaction testing

5.5 Endemic syphilis (A65, A66, A67) – Yaws

Non-endemic countries	Countries where no clinically confirmed and/or serologically confirmed cases have been reported previously to WHO
Endemic countries	Countries where clinically confirmed and/or serologically confirmed cases have been detected and/or reported to WHO
Previously endemic countries	Countries where cases were reported in the past but no cases have been reported to WHO since 1990

5.6 Leprosy (A30)

New cases	Number of newly diagnosed patients reported at the end of each year
New case detection rate	Number of newly diagnosed patients reported at the end of each year/100 000 population
Global number of new cases	Total number of cases reported routinely to WHO by Member States each year.

5.7 Chagas disease (B57)

Global population infected	Estimated number of people who are infected by whichever route of transmission, presented by country
No transmission	No cases of Chagas disease cases and no transmission
Countries without vector transmission	Countries with cases of Chagas disease but without vector transmission
Countries with rare vector transmission	Countries with cases of Chagas disease and with sporadic vector transmission
Countries with active vector transmission	Countries with cases of Chagas disease and with ongoing vector transmission

5.8 Human African trypanosomiasis (B56.0, B56.1)

Global number of new cases	Total number of cases of human African trypanosomiasis officially reported to WHO by each country, each year

5.9 Leishmaniasis (B55.0, B55.1, B55.2)

Endemic areas	Countries in which cases of leishmaniasis have been reported
Free areas	Countries in which cases of leishmaniasis have not been detected or reported

5.10 Cysticercosis (B68.0, B68.1, B69)

No data available	Countries or areas where no reports (published, official, anecdotal) are available. Some countries may not have pigs so no pigs or pork products are consumed; in these countries it would be highly unlikely for the parasite to be present. Other countries may be endemic but no information is available
Imported cases	Countries or areas where imported human cysticercosis cases have been documented as well as some autochthonous cases of cysticercosis in local people who have been infected by "imported" tapeworm carriers from endemic countries, however there is no transmission to pigs either because they are not present or are kept under intensive husbandry systems (e.g., in Europe and the United States)
Suspected endemic	Countries or areas where full life-cycle is suspected to be ongoing (both human and pig infections) based on anecdotal reports, but no formal studies have been undertaken or reported to confirm this
Endemic (full life-cycle)	Countries or areas where people and pigs are infected and the full transmission life-cycle is ongoing (i.e., people with taeniasis transmit cysticercosis to both people and pigs; pigs with cysticercosis transmitting taeniasis to people)

5.11 Dracunculiasis (B72)

Endemic countries	Countries in which a village with 1 or more active indigenous cases have been reported during the previous or current calendar year, or both
Countries in pre-certification stage	Countries where transmission has been interrupted (no indigenous cases present) and an extensive surveillance system for detecting new cases has been sustained for at least three consecutive full years until certification of eradication is granted by WHO
Countries certified	Countries certified as being free of dracunculiasis by WHO on the recommendation of the International Commission for the Certification of Dracunculiasis Eradication

5.12 Cystic echinococcosis (hydatidosis) (B67)

Probably absent	Countries or territories with no confirmed identifications or reports of Echinococcus granulosus in indigenous domestic or wild animal populations. Human cystic echinococcosis (hydatidosis) has not been reported
Suspected	E. granulosus may not be recorded in official data or publications, but may occur in wildlife and possibly at low prevalence in domestic animals. Human cystic echinococcosis (hydatidosis) appears not to occur
Rare/Sporadic	E. granulosus has been recorded at low prevalence in domestic animals and may be transmitted in wildlife populations. Human cystic echinococcosis (hydatidosis) cases are only occasionally reported
Present	E. granulosus is known to be endemic in at least some areas of the country. Domestic animal (and possibly wildlife) and human cystic echinococcosis (hydatidosis) occur regularly
High endemicity areas	The definition applies only to areas within a specified endemic country. High endemicity areas involve ≥1 state, region, province or district where E. granulosus prevalence in dogs exceeds 5-10% and where the prevalence of human cystic echinococcosis (hydatidosis) is greater than 1–5 cases/100 000 inhabitants annually

5.13 Foodborne trematodiasis (B66.0, B66.1, B66.3, B66.4) – fascioliasis

Cases	Actively or passively reported cases of fascioliasis, detected clinically or parasitologically

5.14 Lymphatic filariasis (B74.0, B74.1, B74.2)

Ongoing interventions	Endemic country implementing mass drug administration
Interventions not started	Endemic country that has not commenced implementation of mass drug administration
Interventions stopped after achieving microfilaraemia prevalence rate less than 1%	Endemic country where the microfilaraemia rate has decreased to less than 1% and mass drug administration has been stopped
Not requiring interventions	Historically endemic where no mass drug administration is required
Non-endemic	Country not previously endemic

5.15 Onchocerciasis (B73)

Endemic	Cases of onchocerciasis have been detected previously
Non-endemic	No cases of onchocerciasis have been detected previously

Hypoendemic	Country with onchocercal nodule prevalence rates less than 20% and where individuals are treated on a clinical basis
Mesoendemic	Country with onchocercal nodule prevalence rates of 20–39% and where preventive chemotherapy is required
Hyperendemic	Country with onchocercal nodule prevalence rates greater than 39% and where preventive chemotherapy is required

5.16 Schistosomiasis (B65.0, B65.1, B65.2, B65.8)

Non-endemic	No parasitiologically confirmed cases of schistosomiasis detected or reported.
Low risk of morbidity	Parasitiologically confirmed cases reported, with prevalence less than 10% in affected areas and preventive chemotherapy is not required
Moderate risk of morbidity	Parasitiologically confirmed cases reported, with prevalence of 10% or higher but less than 50% in affected areas and preventive chemotherapy is required
High risk of morbidity	Parasitiologically confirmed cases reported, with prevalence 50% or higher in affected areas and preventive chemotherapy is required

5.17 Soil-transmitted helminthiases (B76.0, B76.1, B77, B79)

Non-endemic	No parasitologically confirmed soil-transmitted helminths reported
Low risk of morbidity	Parasitologically confirmed cases reported, prevalence is less than 20% in affected areas and preventive chemotherapy is not required
Moderate risk of morbidity	Parasitologically confirmed cases reported, with prevalence 20% or higher but less than 50% in affected areas and preventive chemotherapy is required
High risk of morbidity	Parasitologically confirmed cases reported, with prevalence 50% or higher in affected areas and preventive chemotherapy is required

REFERENCES

1. For clinical descriptions and case definitions, see *WHO recommended strategies for the prevention and control of communicable diseases*. Geneva, World Health Organization, 2001 (WHO/CDS/CPE/SMT/2001.13).

2. *International Statistical Classification of Diseases and related health problems*, 10th revision, ICD-10, 2008 edition. Geneva, World Health Organization, 2009.

3. *Trachoma control: a guide for programme managers*. Geneva, World Health Organization, 2006.

Annex 4. Methods used to prepare maps and charts

Population

The total population of each country is taken from *World population prospects: 2009 revision* (*1*). The population of children aged 1–4 years and 5–14 years is also given in some cases since these are the age groups specifically targeted for anthelminthic treatments.

Preventive chemotherapy data

Unless otherwise specified, data on preventive chemotherapy are as provided by national authorities to WHO through reporting processes in country and regional offices using standardized templates. Maps and charts for lymphatic filariasis, soil-transmitted helminthiases, schistosomiasis, onchocerciasis and trachoma were prepared using data routinely reported to WHO annually. Information from the preventive chemotherapy databank was used to compile sections of this report and is accessible online (*2*).

The main definitions of data used to describe preventive chemotherapy are as follows.

> **Population requiring preventive chemotherapy**: the total population living in all endemic areas who require preventive chemotherapy.
>
> **Geographical coverage**: the proportion (%) of endemic districts covered by preventive chemotherapy.
>
> **Programme coverage**: the proportion (%) of individuals who were treated according to the programme's target.
>
> **National disease-specific coverage**: the proportion (%) of individuals in the population requiring preventive chemotherapy for the specific disease that has been treated.

Dracunculiasis data are as reported weekly to WHO by national authorities that provide updates on the status of the eradication initiative at the country level as well as related epidemiological information.

Fascioliasis data are based on information obtained from peer-reviewed publications and supplemented by the opinions of international experts.

Data on innovative and intensified disease management

Data for neglected tropical diseases where the large-scale use of existing tools is limited have been obtained by various non-integrated methods that depend on the particularities of the disease control programme.

> **Chagas disease**: data officially reported to WHO as official estimates endorsed through a consultative process between national authorities and international experts.
>
> **Buruli ulcer**: annual data routinely reported to WHO by national authorities using a standardized reporting template.
>
> **Endemic syphilis**: historical data and ad hoc information reported to WHO by national authorities and researchers.
>
> **Human African trypanosomiasis**: data routinely reported to WHO annually by national authorities using a standardized reporting template.
>
> **Leishmaniasis:** ad hoc information made available to WHO by programme managers and researchers.
>
> **Leprosy:** data routinely reported to WHO annually by national authorities using a standardized reporting template.

Zoonoses data

Rabies: data were obtained from RabNet and other sources. RabNet is a WHO-led interactive information system that is able to generate interactive maps and graphs using data on rabies in humans and animals. This online data collection system collects data electronically on a yearly basis (*3*).

Cysticercosis: data are based on information obtained from peer-reviewed publications and supplemented by the opinions of international experts.

Echinococcosis (hydatidosis): data are based on information obtained from peer-reviewed publications and the opinions of international experts.

Sources of information

Sources of information are as indicated in each diagram and specific chapter. All reasonable precautions have been taken to verify and confirm the accuracy of the information contained in this publication.

REFERENCES

1. *World population prospects: 2008 revision*. New York, NY, United Nations Population Division, 2009.
2. *WHO preventive chemotherapy and transmission control databank*. Geneva, World Health Organization, 2010 (http://www.who.int/neglected_diseases/preventive_chemotherapy/databank/en/index.html; accessed July 2010).
3. *RabNet: human and animal rabies – an interactive and information mapping system* [online database]. Geneva, World Health Organization, 2010 (http://apps.who.int/globalatlas/default.asp).

WHO regional offices

Regional Office for Africa
Cité du Djoué, P.O.Box 06
Brazzaville, Congo
Telephone: + 242 839 100 / +47 241 39100
Facsimile: + 242 839 501 / +47 241 395018
E-mail: regafro@afro.who.int

Regional Office for the Americas
525, 23rd Street, N.W.
Washington, DC 20037, USA
Telephone: +1 202 974 3000
Facsimile: +1 202 974 3663
E-mail: postmaster@paho.org

Regional Office for South-East Asia
World Health House
Indraprastha Estate
Mahatama Gandhi Marg
New Delhi 110 002, India
Telephone: + 91-11-2337 0804
Facsimile: + 91-11-2337 9507
E-mail: guptasmithv@searo.who.int

Regional Office for Europe
8, Scherfigsvej
DK-2100 Copenhagen 0, Denmark
Telephone: + 45 39 171 717
Facsimile: + 45 39 171 818
E-mail: postmaster@euro.who.int

Regional Office for the Eastern Mediterranean
Abdul Razzak Al Sanhouri Street,
P.O. Box 7608,
Nasr City, Cairo 11371, Egypt
Telephone: + 202 2276 50 00
Facsimile: + 202 2670 24 92 or 2670 24 94
E-mail: postmaster@emro.who.int

Regional Office for the Western Pacific
P.O. Box 2932
1000 Manila, Philippines
Telephone: + 63 2 528 8001
E-mail: postmaster@wpro.who.int